D1111828

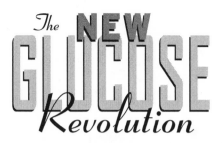

The NEW GLUCOSE Revolution

What Makes My Blood Glucose Go Up . . . and Down?

101 Frequently Asked Questions about Your Blood Glucose Levels

Dr. Jennie Brand-Miller
Kaye Foster-Powell
David Mendosa

MARLOWE & COMPANY
NEW YORK

THE NEW GLUCOSE REVOLUTION
WHAT MAKES MY BLOOD GLUCOSE GO UP . . . AND DOWN?:
101 Frequently Asked Questions about Your Blood Glucose Levels

Copyright © 2003, 2006 by Jennie Brand-Miller,
Kaye Foster-Powell, and David Mendosa

Published by
Marlowe & Company
An Imprint of Avalon Publishing Group, Incorporated
245 West 17th Street • 11th floor
New York, NY 10011

AVALON
publishing group Incorporated

The Library of Congress has cataloged the previous edition as follows:

Brand Miller, Janette, 1952–
What makes my blood glucose go up—and down? : and 101 other frequently asked
questions about your blood glucose levels / Jennie Brand-Miller,
Kaye Foster-Powell, and David Mendosa.
p. cm.
Includes bibliographical references and index.
ISBN 1-56924-574-6
1. Diabetes—Popular works. 2. Blood sugar—Popular works.
3. Hypoglycemia—Popular works. 4. Hyperglycemia—Popular works.
I. Foster-Powell, Kaye. II. Mendosa, David. III. Title.
RC660.4 .B736 2003
616.4'62—dc21   2002038693

ISBN: 1-56924-302-6
ISBN-13: 978-1-56924-302-2

Designed by Pauline Neuwirth, Neuwirth & Associates, Inc
Printed in the United States of America

CONTENTS

PART TWO: WHAT MAKES MY BLOOD GLUCOSE GO UP?

A. Food Factors That Increase My Blood Glucose Levels

INTRODUCTION

What makes my blood glucose (blood sugar) go up . . . and down?

Can you answer that question? Many people wonder about it, some are positively preoccupied by it—particularly those with diabetes. Most of us would say, "Sugar makes my blood glucose rise." That's true, but so does a slice of bread. So does a potato. In fact, a typical potato has nearly twice the effect of two teaspoons of sugar. Surprised? Science has proven that all foods containing carbohydrates will raise your blood glucose level, some more so than others. You can't tell by looking at the food or by studying its composition. Fiber content is no indication and sweetness is no guide either. But knowledge of a food's carbohydrate content and *glycemic load* will help you sort out how common foods affect your blood glucose levels. What's *that* you ask? This book explains it clearly and simply. And at the back of the book, you'll find the glycemic index (GI) and glycemic load (GL) of hundreds of foods.

Foods are not the only cause of high blood glucose levels. Your liver produces glucose too, more so between meals than right after. Emotions, sickness, and hormones can also send your blood glucose levels sky high. Nature makes sure that when it's time to fight or time to fly, there's plenty of fuel available for the purpose.

How do you bring those high glucose levels down? That's easy. You could fast for a few hours. You could get some exercise. You could even do some high-level math. Even if you do nothing, your glucose levels will fall. That's because glucose will eventually move out of the blood and into cells of the body. In the absence of *insulin*, that process is rather slow. Insulin, a powerful hormone, gets things moving quickly by "opening the gates" so that glucose rapidly enters cells and is used as an immediate source of energy.

That answers the first question. Whew . . . only 100 to go. Our goal is to answer all those frequently asked questions about blood glucose—what makes it go up . . . and what makes it go down—and in the process help you to better manage your unpredictable blood glucose levels over the course of a day—day in and day out.

WHO THIS BOOK IS FOR

This book is written for anyone who has ever asked . . .

> *Why are my blood glucose levels so high when I'm doing all the right things?*
> *Why do I need to watch my blood glucose levels—I don't have diabetes?*
> *Are my mood swings related to sugar "highs" and sugar "lows"?*
> *When I feel shaky, is that because my blood glucose levels are low?*
> *Which foods raise my blood glucose levels most?*

We wrote this book for everybody. It's not just for people with diabetes, although they certainly are among those who ask themselves questions like these all the time. The idea for this book arose because every day, in the course of our jobs, we receive questions about blood glucose levels from people all around the world. Some say they have not received satisfactory answers by searching the Internet and libraries. They wonder if we can help. Why, they ask, despite their best efforts, are their blood glucose levels still too high?

We realized that together we had a unique body of knowledge that allowed us to give simple, straightforward answers to virtually any question involving blood glucose levels. We were doing it every day. It was time to make the information more widely available, time to help those who didn't have the time to search the Internet, read widely, or have the expertise to decipher the medical journals themselves.

This book is therefore relevant to many people: those with diabetes, whether type 1 or type 2, and for parents of children with diabetes; it is for those who blame hypoglycemia or low blood glucose levels for their ailments or fatigue; it is for those who want clear, scientifically based information about the connection between food, exercise, weight, and blood glucose levels.

WHAT THIS BOOK COVERS

This book covers 101 questions and answers that range from "What's a normal blood glucose reading?" to "What's a sinful snack I can have that won't raise my blood glucose levels?" They are gleaned from our own experience of the questions people most often ask. Indeed, the majority are actual questions that we've received over the course of the last few years. Our answers are strictly based on the scientific evidence that's available. We don't go out on a limb making claims we can't justify.

There is a logical order to our questions and answers. We start with the simplest ones about the connection between blood glucose levels and health, and then move on to the things that raise blood glucose levels—food, stress, illness—and finally to the things that lower our blood glucose levels. Along the way, we explore the intricacies of the glycemic index of foods, the effects of fat and protein, fiber, and herbs and spices. To keep things as simple as possible, all terms that appear in **boldface** in the text are defined in the glossary at the end of the book. We leave no stone unturned.

We've given you the answers that you can't find anywhere else.

WHY WE WROTE THIS BOOK

We wrote this book first and foremost because of the amazing curiosity of our readers. We were surprised and pleased to find that so many of them wanted scientific explanations for the way things were. Why did one food make blood glucose levels high and another food not affect them at all? Why did they have higher blood glucose levels in the morning than before bed? They hadn't eaten anything in their sleep as far as they were aware!

One of the reasons people have so many questions is that there's a lot of confusion out there. Nearly every day the media focuses attention on yet another diet, one more expert who contradicts another. But hey, controversy sells newspapers, doesn't it? In truth, science and medicine can now answer most of the questions related to food, blood glucose levels, and health.

We were driven to write this book because it never ceases to amaze us how thoughtful and intelligent people are with their questions. It was obvious they want answers, but ones that don't baffle and confuse, ones couched in language they can comprehend, not steeped in medical and scientific obfuscation.

We feel that a small book that puts all these questions and answers together might be just what the doctor ordered.

WHO WE ARE

Jennie Brand-Miller is Professor of Human Nutrition at the University of Sydney, Australia's first and foremost university. She is the current president of the Nutrition Society of Australia and is one of the authors of *The New Glucose Revolution* and many other titles in the Glucose Revolution series. She has taught postgraduate students of nutrition and dietetics at the University of Sydney for over twenty-four years, and currently leads a team of twelve research scientists whose interests focus on all aspects of carbohydrates— diet and diabetes, the glycemic index of foods, insulin resistance, lactose intolerance, and oligosaccharides in infant nutrition. She holds a special interest in evolutionary nutrition and the diet of Australian Aborigines. Jennie has published sixteen books and 150 journal articles.

Kaye Foster-Powell is an accredited practicing dietitian with extensive experience in diabetes management. A graduate of the University of Sydney (B.Sc., Master of Nutrition and Dietetics), she has conducted research into the glycemic index of foods and its practical implications over the last fifteen years. She has coauthored all the books in the Glucose Revolution series and published the International Tables of Glycemic Index, the first compilation of glycemic index values of foods from around the world. She is currently a dietitian with Wentworth Area Diabetes Service in Sydney, and provides consultancy to health professionals and the general public on all aspects of the glycemic index.

David Mendosa is a freelance journalist and consultant specializing in diabetes. After earning a B.A. with honors from the University of California, Riverside, and an M.A. from Claremont Graduate University, he became a Foreign Service officer. He worked eleven years in Washington and four years in Africa for the U.S. foreign aid program. Subsequently, he became a journalist, initially specializing in writing about small business. But when he was diagnosed with type 2 diabetes in February 1994, he began to write entirely about that condition. His articles and columns have appeared in many of the major diabetes magazines and Web sites. His own Web site, David Mendosa's Diabetes Directory, www.mendosa.com/diabetes.htm, was one of the first and is now one of the largest with that focus. He also publishes a monthly online newsletter called "Diabetes Update."

Together, the three of us make a rare and great combination—the scientist, the practical dietitian, and the realist with diabetes. What more could you ask for?! So read on, you'll be truly amazed.

PART

1

Your Blood Glucose Levels

1. What is a normal blood glucose level?

If you haven't eaten in the past few hours, the normal blood **glucose** level falls within the range 60 to 110 milligrams per deciliter (mg/dl). Upon eating, the level will rise, but rarely beyond 180 mg/dl. The extent of the rise will vary, depending on your individual physiological response (your glucose "tolerance") and the type of food you've eaten. Although blood glucose levels fluctuate over the course of a day, they will normally remain within this fairly narrow range. We can thank two hormones for this—**insulin** and **glucagon**—which finely regulate the level of glucose in our blood.

Carbohydrates in food are responsible for most of the rise in glucose that occurs after a meal. Digestion of carbohydrates actually begins in the mouth, where saliva acts on starch. It continues in the stomach and small intestine until all the starches and sugars have been broken down into their simplest forms—the "mono" sugars: glucose, **fructose**, and **galactose**—and absorbed across the wall of the intestine into the blood stream.

The presence of glucose in the blood triggers rapid secretion of insulin from the pancreas. Insulin causes uptake, storage, and use of glucose by the cells of the body. About half of the glucose absorbed after a meal is stored as **glycogen** in the muscles and liver. Between meals, when blood glucose levels start to fall, the hormone glucagon triggers the release of this stored sugar. The liver also makes *new* glucose molecules when it needs to, using the body's fat and protein stores. The body has mechanisms that stop blood glucose levels from falling too low, even when you go without food for a long time.

Most people with diabetes have a relative lack of insulin, and consequently their blood glucose levels tend to be higher. The American Diabetes Association recommends levels in the range of 80–120 mg/dl before meals and 100–140 mg/dl at bedtime. Keeping levels within the normal range is important whether you have diabetes or not.

KEEPING THOSE HORMONES STRAIGHT . . .

Insulin: A hormone produced by the pancreas that works to bring blood glucose levels down. It does this by "opening the gates" of cells and moving glucose from the bloodstream into the body cells. It also switches off the synthesis of any new glucose by the liver and the breakdown of fat as a source of energy.

Glucagon: Another hormone produced by the pancreas that has the opposite effect to insulin. It causes blood glucose levels to rise by getting the liver to release some of its glucose stores and to make new glucose to release into the blood.

Figure 1. Normal blood glucose levels before and after a meal.

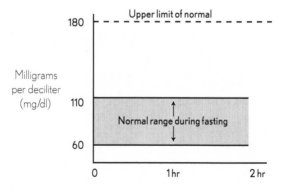

LOW, MEDIUM, AND
HIGH BLOOD GLUCOSE LEVELS

Most of the time our blood glucose levels fluctuate between 60-110mg/dl. They rise after a meal, but return to the normal range within one to two hours in a person with normal glucose tolerance. This picture illustrates low (20-50mg/dl), normal (60-110mg/dl), and high (above 200mg/dl) blood glucose levels for people with diabetes.

Figure 2. Low, normal, and high blood glucose ranges in the fasting state (i.e., before breakfast).

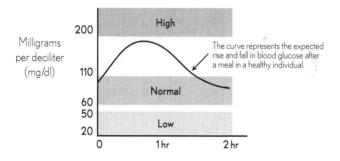

2. What's wrong with a high blood glucose level?

High blood glucose levels pose a concealed threat to our health. Long before we know they are high, and before diabetes would be diagnosed, moderately elevated blood glucose levels damage our heart and circulatory system. They increase our risk of a heart attack, **type 2 diabetes**, weight gain, and possibly certain types of cancer. In fact, research is showing that moderately elevated blood glucose levels have a far greater impact on our body than we could ever have imagined (see question 7).

When someone has high blood glucose levels over time (as can happen in people with diabetes) the effects on the body become more noticeable. Problems may occur with the skin so that bacterial infections, fungal infections, and itching are more common. Nerves may be damaged so that numbness, prickling, tingling, burning, and aching sensations are experienced. There may be a loss of nerve function so that a process like digestion is impaired. The narrowing of large blood vessels will slow blood flow and cause heart disease, stroke, and loss of circulation, which may lead to amputation. There also may be damage to small blood vessels, which can cause problems ranging from blurry vision to blindness or kidney disease.

Very high blood glucose levels (above 360 mg/dl) that can occur in those with diabetes can be life-threatening if left untreated. Levels this high reflect a lack of insulin in the body, meaning that glucose cannot be used for fuel. As an alternative, our body breaks down fats for energy. With the breakdown of fat, the release of fatty acids into the blood can be so high that the body can't burn them fast enough.

When this happens, by-products called **ketones** or keto-acids build up in the blood stream and disturb the body's acid-base balance. A condition known as **ketoacidosis** develops, which requires immediate medical attention.

3. What's wrong with a low blood glucose level?

As we described earlier, our blood glucose levels are finely regulated within a fairly narrow operating range. One reason for this is to ensure a critical level of glucose to provide energy for our brains. The brain is the most energy-demanding organ in our body—responsible for over half of our obligatory fuel requirements. And unlike other body organs, our brain relies almost exclusively on glucose as a source of fuel. Any shortfall in glucose availability therefore has consequences for brain function.

In the most severe case, when blood glucose levels are in the range of 20 to 50 mg/dl, we develop **hypoglycemia**. If this occurs you might feel confused, shaky, dizzy, sweaty, or have a headache, tingling around the lips, pale skin, or make clumsy or jerky movements. Treat the symptoms by having glucose tabs or glucose gel if you can. But if your level goes so low that you are unconscious, a person trained in injecting glucagon can give you a shot from a Glucagon Emergency Kit. Everyone who uses insulin should have one of these kits on hand at all times. In the United States, they are dispensed by prescription only. Your body will usually respond in five to 10 minutes, but if not, your caregiver must call an ambulance or rush you to a hospital.

Mildly reduced blood glucose levels impair mental performance too, although to a lesser extent. Recent medical literature shows that performance of demanding mental tasks and "intelligence" tests, such as word recall, maze learning, and arithmetic, is improved following the intake of glucose or carbohydrate-rich food. Furthermore, blood glucose levels decline more during a period of intense cognitive processing. This means arithmetic uses up more glucose than simple tasks like reading a magazine. All in all, the evidence points to the importance of a normal blood glucose level for optimal health and performance.

4. How long does it take for my blood glucose to go up after I eat?

The digestion of carbohydrates from foods begins in the mouth. Consequently, glucose levels can rise rapidly after eating. Within fifteen minutes of eating we can measure an increase in blood glucose levels of around 36 mg/dl. Levels continue to rise, generally reaching a peak in around thirty to forty-five minutes (although this varies considerably depending on the timing, quantity, and composition of your meal) and by three to four hours the blood glucose has returned to pre-meal levels. In people with diabetes, the peak is delayed to around one hour after the start of the meal, and the return to pre-meal levels can take much longer. That's not to say that all the carbohydrates in a meal will have been digested and absorbed by then. Some slowly digested forms of carbohydrate take over four or five hours to be completely absorbed—that's why foods like lentils make you feel fuller for longer. In fact, all legumes have this effect of slow and extended absorption. Because the rate of absorption is so slow, blood glucose levels are only slightly elevated in the hours following their consumption.

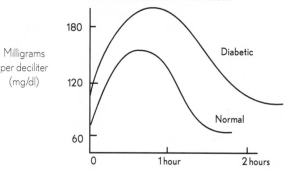

Figure 3. Blood glucose levels before and after a meal in a normal and diabetic individual.

5. What is the best time to test my blood glucose?

To keep an eye on your blood glucose levels, it is advisable to do some regular fasting tests—first thing in the morning before you've had anything to eat or drink—and some tests two hours after you first begin to eat a meal. How much testing you want to do is your decision. Testing once a day, at varying times—for example, a fasting test on one day, two hours after breakfast the next day, two hours after lunch the following day, etc.—is a commonly recommended regime. We suggest that you discuss the most appropriate times to test your blood glucose levels with your doctor.

When you test, you will need your own blood glucose meter and the test strips that work with that meter. These meters are often available, at little cost, at local or online drugstores. Many diabetes educators and doctors give out free blood glucose meters. However, the test strips can get expensive if you test regularly. We suggest that you get a prescription from your doctor for a meter and supplies covered by your health insurance provider, if you have one. In almost all states, health insurance plans are required to offer coverage for at least one brand. You can check http://www.diabetes.org/main/community/advocacy/states2.jsp to see what your state requires. For a complete directory of the meters on the market now in the United States, see http://www.mendosa.com/meters.htm.

6. Why has my doctor asked me to test before meals?

Generally, your doctor would only ask you to test before meals to check the effectiveness of your diabetes medication or insulin. Normally, it's advisable to ensure that you test at least two hours since you last ate. Even snacks between meals must be counted. A pre-meal test will show if your blood glucose level has come back down to baseline or whether your glucose is running too high or too low in-between the meals. This feedback regarding the action of your last dose of insulin or medication can help the doctor decide what and when your next dose should be. If your blood glucose levels are low at this time, it's important to reduce your insulin or medication dose so that you don't run the risk of hypoglycemia. If your blood glucose is too high, your doctor may want to prescribe a higher dose or a longer-acting form of insulin or medication.

7. I don't have diabetes. Do I still need to watch my blood glucose levels?

Blood glucose levels can still be too high, even if you don't have diabetes. In fact, for every three people with diabetes, there is one who has it but doesn't know it. There are also many people whose blood glucose levels are not in the diabetic range but are still high enough to be a health risk. About 16 million American adults have this condition, referred to as **pre-diabetes**. It is often present as part of the syndrome called **Syndrome X**, which is also referred to as "the metabolic syndrome" or "insulin resistance syndrome."

People with pre-diabetes have difficulty bringing their blood glucose levels back to normal after consuming a meal containing carbohydrates and/or have elevated blood glucose levels after fasting. Pre-diabetes is officially diagnosed when either the fasting (before breakfast) blood glucose reading is between 110 and 126 mg/dl or when glucose levels after an oral glucose tolerance test are between 140 and 200 mg/dl.

So what's so undesirable about this? In practice, it means that every meal is a stress to the body, particularly the walls lining the blood vessels. Blood glucose levels in this range are "toxic," causing a series of undesirable reactions. Excess glucose in the blood acts as a powerful oxidizing agent, producing compounds called "free radicals" that in turn oxidize other compounds, including fats in the blood. Oxidized fats are far more harmful than normal fats, increasing the risk of hardened artery walls. High blood pressure develops. High blood glucose levels also increase the tendency of blood to form clots, increasing the chance of heart attack.

High blood glucose levels also increase the formation of products called "advanced glycated endproducts" or AGEs. As the name implies, these substances are associated with aging, including sagging of the skin and the slowing down of all cellular reactions. Even Alzheimer's has been associated with deposits of AGEs in the brain.

Lastly, it's known that high blood glucose levels (and the accompanying high insulin levels) increase the risk of becoming overweight and/or developing type 2 diabetes. The upshot of all this is that high blood glucose levels should be a concern to many people, but only a small fraction will know they have them. Ask your doctor to measure your glucose levels the next time you visit.

SYNDROME X
THE METABOLIC SYNDROME
INSULIN RESISTANCE SYNDROME

Do you have . . .

High blood pressure?
Impaired glucose tolerance or diabetes?
High blood fats (triglycerides)?
Excess fat around your middle?
Low HDL (good) cholesterol levels?

If you answer "yes" to more than two of these, chances are you have syndrome X, also known as the metabolic syndrome or insulin resistance syndrome. This condition is characterized by a collection of metabolic abnormalities that greatly increase the chance of heart attack.

8. I have terrible mood swings. Could that have anything to do with my blood glucose levels?

Mood swings are not normally related to rises and falls in blood glucose. They are not a classical symptom of diabetes, nor is there evidence that people with diabetes are more susceptible to mood changes than others. When a person with diabetes experiences very low blood glucose, however, brain function is impaired (see question 3), which may appear like a change in mood.

What's more, rapid rises and falls in blood glucose do cause "stress" to the body. That stress is sufficient to elicit the production of stress hormones such as glucagon and **cortisol**. Thus, the body is in "flight-or-fight" mode after a rapid rise and fall in blood glucose levels. This effect has been demonstrated even in healthy young people. In susceptible individuals dramatic falls in blood glucose levels could be associated with tremor, nausea, or dizziness. Some people refer to a "sugar high" and a "sugar low" after consuming sugary foods, but this is unlikely to have anything to do with blood glucose levels. If it was, they would experience the same feelings after eating starchy foods like rice, bread, and potatoes, because these foods raise blood glucose just as much—if not more than—sugary foods. See question 45 for further discussion on sugar's impact.

Some women have told us that their severe symptoms of premenstrual tension resolved after adopting a diet designed to reduce blood glucose fluctuations (see question 61 for more details about low **glycemic index** diets). But it's important to say that there's no scientific evidence at this point to back up this particular claim.

9. What are the factors that affect my blood glucose level?

Carbohydrates in our diet are the main source of the glucose in our blood, but there are many other factors in addition to food that affect our blood glucose levels.

- The time of day. Blood glucose levels are commonly higher in the morning. We discuss the reason for this in question 60.
- Emotional Stress. Intense emotional stress triggers the release of adrenaline as a part of the body's "fight-or-flight" response. This stimulates glucose release from the liver to increase the availability of glucose to the muscles, so you will see a rise in your blood glucose levels.
- Infection. You may just have a cold developing or a sore that isn't healing, but either way, your body is in defense mode and tries to keep glucose in the blood as fuel to fight infection. Interestingly, an increase in your blood glucose level may precede the onset of other symptoms.
- Pain and surgery. Physical pain increases your blood glucose level through the effect of stress and counter-regulatory hormones.
- Intense heat and cold. These are both physical stressors that can increase the body's **insulin resistance** and raise blood glucose levels.
- A hot shower or bath increases peripheral blood flow and can have a glucose lowering effect.
- Your level of activity. Usually, the more physical activity you do, the lower your blood glucose levels will be. There are exceptions, however, if the activity has been

too stressful or your sugar levels were too high to begin with (see question 95).

‣ Menstrual cycle. Blood glucose levels can vary depending on the stage of your menstrual cycle.

‣ Pregnancy. Blood glucose levels will usually rise during pregnancy.

‣ Your testing technique. If you are using a meter to test your blood glucose levels, are you using it correctly and at the most appropriate time? Perhaps it's time to check its accuracy. Is it correctly calibrated? When did you last run a control solution through it? How fresh are your test strips? Are they within the "use by" date, and have they been correctly stored? Are your hands clean and free of soap or hand cream that might affect the result?

‣ Alcohol. Alcohol reduces glucose released by the liver, which can result in lower blood glucose levels many hours after consuming it.

10. What effect do medications have on blood glucose levels?

Diabetes medications work to lower blood glucose levels. There are many types available. These are discussed in more detail in question 96.

Other medications can also affect the body's blood glucose control. Whenever your doctor prescribes new medications and you have diabetes, it is worthwhile asking, "How will this affect my blood glucose level?" Monitor your blood glucose levels more closely when you change the type or dosage of your medication.

Common drugs which may *increase* your blood glucose levels:
- Beta blockers
- Calcium channel blockers
- Furosemide
- Thiazide diuretics
- Corticosteroids

Common drugs which may *decrease* your blood glucose levels:
- angiotensin converting enzyme (ACE) inhibitors
- Alpha blockers
- Estrogen (high dose)
- Fibric acid derivatives (clofibrate)
- Anabolic steroids
- Salicylates (high dose)

11. What's the difference between complex carbohydrates and simple carbohydrates?

The terms simple and complex carbohydrates were originally coined to differentiate between sugary and starchy foods, based on the chemical structure of the carbohydrate they contained. Sugars were simple and starches were complex, simply because sugars were small molecules and starches were big. By virtue of their large size, it was assumed that complex carbohydrates were more slowly digested and absorbed, and caused a small and gradual rise in blood glucose levels. Sugars, on the other hand, were assumed to be digested rapidly, causing a large rise in blood glucose levels.

Complex carbohydrates are also used to describe starchy foods such as potatoes, bread, rice, pasta, legumes, and breakfast cereals. Simple carbohydrates refers to sugars, as found in soft drinks, candy, ice cream, cookies, cakes, and fruit.

STARCHY FOODS, SUGARY FOODS
—WHAT'S THE DIFFERENCE?

Sugar and starch are both carbohydrates.

Starches are found in foods like potato, rice, and bread.

Sugars are found in foods like table sugar, honey, fruit, milk, and candy.

Starches consist of chains of glucose molecules joined together.

Sugars consist of one glucose molecule joined to either fructose or galactose.

The chemical structure does not determine the rate of digestion of the carbohydrate.

We now know that the whole concept of simple versus complex carbohydrates does not tell us anything about how foods affect our blood glucose levels, and that the assumptions about the speed of digestion were all wrong. It wasn't until the 1980s that scientists studied the actual blood glucose responses to a range of common foods and developed a new system for describing the nature of carbohydrates and classifying them according to their effects on blood glucose levels—the glycemic index (see question 14).

Figure 4. The chemical structures of starch and sugars.

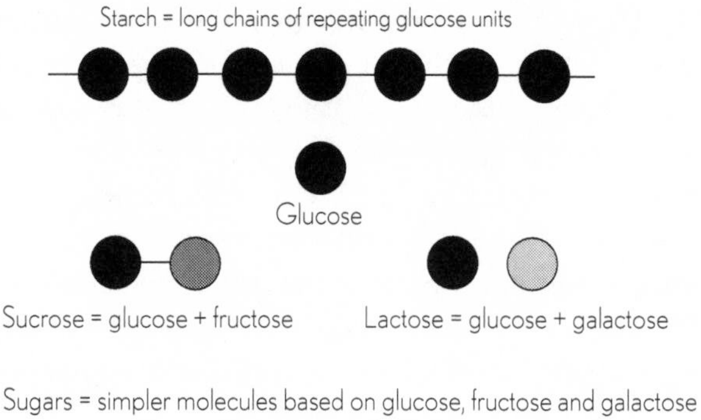

Starch = long chains of repeating glucose units

Glucose

Sucrose = glucose + fructose   Lactose = glucose + galactose

Sugars = simpler molecules based on glucose, fructose and galactose

12. How much carbohydrate should a person eat at one sitting?

It depends on your overall calorie intake. If you are an average-weight man or woman who is moderately active, then your carbohydrate intake at one sitting should be about 60 grams per meal and 30 grams per snack. This amounts to half of your calories as carbohydrate, a level that is considered healthy. If you'd prefer to eat less carbohydrate in favor of a little more protein and unsaturated fat, then you should aim for 50 grams of carbohydrate per meal and 25 grams per snack. This gives you 40 percent of your calories as carbohydrates. Authorities do not recommend lower carbohydrate intake for reasons we've outlined in the answer to Question 68.

If you are overweight and trying to lose some of that excess body fat, then we recommend you still aim for about 45 grams of carbohydrate per meal with 10–15 grams per snack. This gives you a relatively high carbohydrate intake as a proportion of total calories. It's important, however, to choose the right kind of carbohydrate.

If you are an active person engaged in vigorous activity on most days, then you should raise your carbohydrates at mealtime to 75 grams, with snacks containing 30 to 40 grams of carbohydrate.

Whatever your appropriate intake level, we recommend that you eat about half of your carbs in a high-fiber, slowly digested, or whole-grain form. This ensures optimum **insulin sensitivity** and maximum **satiety**—your best path to sensible weight and appetite control.

HOW MUCH CARBOHYDRATE
IS RIGHT FOR YOU?

This table shows recommended carbohydrate servings for adults with different energy needs. It assumes three meals and two or three snacks per day.

	Carbohydrate at 40% of total energy	Carbohydrate at 50% of total energy
Average weight, moderately active adult (1900 cal)	50 grams per meal 15–25 grams per snack	60 grams per meal 20–30 grams per snack
Overweight and trying to lose (1200 cal)	35 grams per meal 15 grams per snack	45 grams per meal 10–15 grams per snack
Average weight, vigorously active adult (2500 cal)	65 grams per meal 20–30 grams per snack	75 grams per meal 30–40 grams per snack

13. How can I find the carbohydrate content of a food that doesn't have a nutrition label?

The Agriculture Research Service of the U.S. Department of Agriculture has the best free resource. It's called the USDA Nutrient Database for Standard Reference, Release 15. It provides data on 6,220 foods for up to 117 nutrients and food components.

This database is available online. The address is http://www.nal.usda.gov/fnic/cgi-bin/nut_search.pl.

Suppose you wanted to know the carbohydrate content of zucchini. Type that word into the search box. It gives you a choice of zucchini in eight forms (including cooked, raw, canned, and frozen). Let's choose it cooked without salt and then choose 1 cup as the size. It shows that 1 cup of zucchini contains 7.1 grams of carbohydrate. The catch is that in the United States, measures of carbohydrate include dietary fiber. But dietary fiber is indigestible, and has no effect on blood glucose, so we need to subtract the fiber figure to give us only the carbohydrate that is available for digestion. In our zucchini example, the fiber content is 2.5 grams, so subtracting this from 7.1 leaves 4.6 grams of available carbohydrate per cup of cooked zucchini.

If you don't have Internet access, the USDA Nutrient Database for Standard Reference, Release 14 is available on CD-ROM from the Government Printing Office. Write to:

Superintendent of Documents
PO Box 371954
Pittsburgh, PA 15250-7954
Stock Number: 001-000-04699-3; Price is $21.00 (U.S.) and $29.40 (non-U.S.).

These databases are the successor to Agriculture Handbook No. 8, Composition of Foods, which is out of print.

There are also books that build on the USDA database. The food composition "bible" is Bowes & Church's *Food Values of Portions Commonly Used*. The current 17th edition lists for $49.95 and covers 8,500 foods.

14. What is the glycemic index?

The glycemic index, or GI, is a numerical way of describing the *type* of carbohydrate in foods according to how it affects blood glucose levels—its glycemic potency. Remember that "glycemic" simply means *glucose in the blood*. The GI value is a measure of carbohydrate *quality*, not quantity. Foods are ranked on the GI scale from 0 to 100, where pure glucose has a rating of 100. Gram for gram of carbohydrate, foods with a high-GI value (70 and over) have more effect than foods with a low-GI (55 or less). Readers familiar with carbohydrate exchanges can think of the glycemic index as a ranking of exchanges according to their true effects on blood glucose levels.

The GI value is determined by feeding equal carbohydrate portions (usually 25 or 50 grams, but any amount can be tested) to a group of eight to ten people and comparing the blood glucose response to their individual responses to the same amount of carbohydrate as pure glucose. If spaghetti shows on average only 40 percent of the glycemic effect of pure glucose, then its GI value is 40. See question 15 on the next page for more information on measuring GI values.

At the back of this book you'll find the GI values for hundreds of foods, all based on real-life testing. If you'd like to read more about the GI of foods and how to put it into practice, *The New Glucose Revolution* (Marlowe & Company, 2003) and its associated pocket guides are the best resources available.

15. How do scientists measure the glycemic index values of foods?

The GI values of foods must be tested in real human beings, not test tubes. A group of eight to ten people are asked to consume a serving of the food within a ten to fifteen-minute period. The size of the serving must contain a standard amount of available carbohydrate—usually it's 50 grams (but it could be 10 or 20 or 30 grams, etc.). A sample of capillary blood is taken from the fingertips just before the meal and then every fifteen minutes for the next hour, and every thirty minutes for the second hour, and measured for glucose concentration.

Analysis of the glucose in the blood shows that the blood glucose concentration rises soon after the start of the meal, reaches a peak at about thirty to forty-five minutes, and then usually falls back to baseline levels within two to three hours. In some cases, it falls below baseline. The results are then graphed on a computer, and what researchers refer to as the "area under the curve" is calculated (see figure 5).

On another occasion, the same volunteers consume the same quantity of carbohydrate in pure glucose—the reference food—and the procedure is repeated. By definition, the reference food has a GI value of 100. In each individual, the area under the curve for the test food is expressed as a percentage of the area under curve for the reference food. The average for the whole group is the GI value of the food. The amount tested is irrelevant—the glycemic index is the glycemic potency of each gram of carbohydrate in a food.

The final values are equally applicable to people with or without diabetes. Studies have shown that the same food tested in two different groups will yield the same result, as long as the standard method is followed. Will the findings be different in people with diabetes? No—it makes little or no difference if the subjects are overweight or have diabetes. Different individuals have their own unique glycemic profile (it will be higher in people with diabetes), and the fact that the test food is compared to a reference food in each and every individual keeps everything relative.

Figure 5. Measuring the glycemic index of foods.

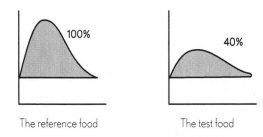

The reference food   The test food

In each individual, the area under the curve corresponding to the test food is expressed as a percentage of that shown for the reference food—pure glucose. In each case, the amount of carbohydrate consumed must be the same.

16. Can I measure the GI value of a food myself?

Calculating the glycemic index of a food requires teams of volunteers to test the result of that food compared with a reference food (like white bread or glucose) on a number of occasions, over a period of several days. Their blood glucose levels are tested at regular intervals for several hours after they eat the test and reference foods, so that the overall rise in their blood glucose, rather than just one or two peaks, is measured.

All this makes it extremely difficult for you to measure the GI value of a food yourself. Even if you were to test your blood glucose several times after eating the food in question and compare those results with a reference food, many other factors can affect your individual response. These include stress, the time of day, recent exercise, your health, and how long it was since your previous meal. What you find may not be representative. On the other hand, the published GI values will be indicative of your *average* result.

This doesn't mean you shouldn't test your blood glucose after a meal—just realize that a two-hour reading will not necessarily reflect the GI value of the food you are eating. The latest guidelines of professional diabetes organizations recommend that you regularly test two hours after beginning a meal, at which point your blood glucose should be at a level below 140 mg/dl.

17. Can you tell me what the range is for low, medium, and high on the GI scale?

A high-GI value is 70 or more, a medium-GI value is 56 to 69 inclusive, and a low-GI is 55 or less. These are the ranges given in *The New Glucose Revolution* and are based on practical experience using the glycemic index.

These ranges are also used in the Glycemic Index Symbol Program in Australia. This program is run by Glycemic Index Limited, a nonprofit company whose members are the University of Sydney, Diabetes Australia, and the Juvenile Diabetes Research Foundation. Currently, foods marketed in Australia can be licensed to become part of the Glycemic Index Symbol Program if they meet strict nutritional criteria and have been properly tested. The trademark is also registered in North America and the United Kingdom, but there are no products carrying the symbol in these locations at the present time.

Does this mean that you should completely avoid high-GI foods? That's not necessary. Instead, focus on lowering the overall GI value of your diet by substituting some low-GI foods for high-GI value foods. When you do eat high-GI value foods, eat less of them than you did before, but don't restrict your food choices unnecessarily.

HIGH, MEDIUM, OR LOW GI?

High GI	70 or more
Baked Russet potatoes	85
Cornflakes	81
Shredded wheat	75
Cheerios™	74
Popcorn	72
Watermelon	72
Whole wheat flour bread	71
White wheat flour bread	70

Medium GI	56–69
Sucrose (table sugar)	68
Life™ cereal	66
Couscous	65
Cantaloupe	65
Beets	64
White rice	64
Sweet potatoes	61
Pineapple	59
New potatoes	57
Wild rice	57

Low GI	55 or less
Buckwheat	54
Sourdough wheat bread	54
Sweet corn	54
Bananas	52
Linguine	52
Orange juice	50

Carrots	47
Parboiled rice	47
Macaroni	47
Grapes	46
Oranges	42
Peaches	42
Spaghetti	42
All-bran cereal	42
Apple juice	40
Strawberries	40
Fettucine	40
Pinto beans	39
Apples	38
Pears	38
Navy beans	38
Kidney beans	28
Chick peas	28
Red lentils	26
Pearled barley	25
Peanuts	14
Chana dal	8
Nopal	7

18. Are foods with lower GI values better than those with higher ones?

If you are comparing like with like, yes. If you are comparing one bread with another or one breakfast cereal with another, generally, the lower the better. But that's not the whole story—the GI value of a food doesn't give us any picture of the food's other nutritional merits or pitfalls. For example, a high-GI food may be a better source of fiber, or lower in salt. Some low-GI foods contain too much saturated fat, too much salt, too many calories, or in other ways may be poor choices for your individual needs. It may also be important to consider the amount of food that you eat and its **glycemic load** (see question 29).

Under certain circumstances, high-GI foods may be the better choice. Athletes, for example, can perform better and replenish their glycogen stores more efficiently after exercise with a food containing glucose that is absorbed more quickly. A high carbohydrate sports drink, a bowl of cornflakes, or a sandwich would be suitable examples.

A single number cannot measure the value of any food, but a single number *can* tell you a great deal about how the carbohydrate in that food affects blood glucose levels. High blood glucose levels are a risk factor for diabetes and cardiovascular disease. Dozens of studies have shown improvements in these levels when people follow low-GI diets.

19. What do you mean by "available" carbohydrate?

When we talk about available carbohydrate, we mean all carbohydrate except that which escapes digestion in the small intestine. The escapees include fiber, some sugars and sugar alcohols, and very small amounts of starch that resists digestion. Available carbohydrate is the carbohydrate that can be absorbed into the bloodstream. Some people refer to it as "glycemic" or "usable" or "net" carbohydrate. These terms refer to the same thing.

Many countries, including the United States and Canada, determine the amount of carbohydrate in foods indirectly, that is "by difference." They measure the protein, fat, water, and ash per 100 grams and subtract the sum of these from 100. In contrast, countries in Europe and Oceania analyze carbohydrate content directly, so their carbohydrate figures do not contain unavailable carbohydrate (e.g., fiber), while values for the United States and Canada do.

As a result of this international difference, nutrition labels on packages imported to the U.S. from Europe and Oceania can be misinterpreted. For example, Bran–A–Crisp Fiber Bread, from Norway, is sold in the United States with a nutrition label that says it has 6 grams of carbohydrates and 6 grams of fiber. It would be a mistake to conclude that this product contains no available carbohydrate. By comparison, Lavosh crisp bread made in America says on its nutrition label that it has 24.8 grams of carbohydrate per serving and 1.1 grams of dietary fiber. Since it follows U.S. practice, the fiber is included in the carbohydrate, so this crisp bread actually has 23.7 grams of "available" carbohydrate per serving.

20. If testing continued for long enough, wouldn't I end up with the same amount of glucose in my blood, even from very high-GI and very low-GI foods?

Many people make the assumption that since the amount of carbohydrate in the test portions of food is the same, then the total amount of glucose in the blood must eventually work out to be the same. However, this is not the case, because the body is not only absorbing glucose from the gut into the bloodstream, it is simultaneously *extracting* glucose from the blood.

Just as gentle rain can be taken up by the garden better than a sudden deluge, the body can metabolize slowly absorbed glucose more easily. Fast-release carbohydrate causes "flooding" of glucose into the bloodstream. Just as water levels in the river rise quickly after torrential rain, so do glucose levels in the blood when a high-GI food is ingested. The metabolic machinery simply cannot extract glucose from the blood fast enough.

Figure 6. Heavy rain causes flooding and dam levels rise, while gentle rain is good for the garden. A flood of glucose into the blood stream overwhelms the body's ability to dispose of glucose, so glucose levels rise. But a slow trickle of glucose can be almost imperceptible and is good for health.

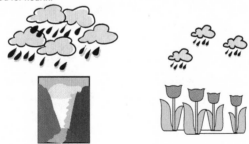

But if a slow and steady amount of rain falls over a longer period, it can be absorbed into the ground and water levels, or blood glucose levels, remain under control. And so it is with low-GI foods.

21. What size portion does the GI value of a food relate to? Say the GI value for bananas is 55—does this value correspond to one banana? If so, what is the size of the banana, big or small?

A food's glycemic index (GI) value does not refer to a specific quantity of food. Rather, the GI is a measure that reflects the *quality* or *nature* of the carbohydrate in that food—specifically, its ability to raise blood glucose levels. It compares one unit of carbohydrate in a food with the *same* unit of carbohydrate in another food, or one carbohydrate exchange with another. Those of us who are fond of diamonds will be familiar with the fact that diamonds are not all the same. A one-carat diamond can vary in price because of differences in its color, brilliance, clarity, etc. So it is with the carbohydrates in food—they have different glycemic effects for the same weight of carbohydrate.

For this reason, the best way to use the glycemic index is to switch from a high-GI to a low-GI food within the same food category. One slice of regular white bread has about the same carbohydrate content as 100 percent whole grain bread, but their GI values vary significantly (70 versus 35). Similarly, a serving of long grain boiled rice will have much the same carbohydrate content as long grain quick-cooking rice, but the GI values vary by about fifteen units (56 versus 75).

The answer to the question, then, is that the GI value of a banana is the same whatever the size of the banana. What changes, however, with increasing serving size is the total glycemic response to the banana. The *total* glycemic response—which we call the glycemic load— is determined by *both* the carbohydrate quantity and quality. We show you how to compare blood glucose levels after servings of food that vary in both carbohydrate content and glycemic index in the answer to question 31.

22. If the glycemic index of a food is the same no matter how much I eat, does it matter if I eat more or less? If I eat twice as much, will my blood glucose level double?

Yes, it does matter how much you eat! Up to a point, the more you eat, the higher your blood glucose level will be. We say "up to a point" because blood glucose levels don't continue to rise indefinitely, thanks to the secretion of insulin. If you eat twice as much, your blood glucose level is unlikely to double, but the demand for insulin will. So why does the GI value matter? Well, the lower the glycemic index, the more you can eat before your blood glucose rises too high.

23. How can I find out what a food's GI value is?

We now know the GI value of more than 750 different types of foods. These can be found in the glycemic index tables in the back of this book. You can also look up the GI value of a food online at www.glycemicindex.com. On the home page, just click on the searchable GI database. When the window pops up, type the name of the food you wish to look up. Click "Go" and the GI value of all the foods containing that word will appear (e.g., if you typed in apple, you'll get the GI value of an apple, apple muffin, apple pie, etc.). The amount of carbohydrate per nominal serving and the calculated glycemic load (GI value × carbohydrate per serving/100) will also be shown. This online database is updated every month.

You can also find the glycemic index and glycemic loads of these foods at www.mendosa.com/gilists.htm, the end of this book, or in *The New Glucose Revolution*.

A small but increasing number of foods have the GI value on the label. Australian food manufacturers lead the world in this respect. This has been made possible through an accredited glycemic index testing program conducted through the University of Sydney. We believe that knowledge of the GI value of foods is becoming increasingly important to the population and encourage people to write and call food manufacturers asking them to have their favorite foods tested. The site, www.gisymbol.com, provides information about the glycemic index testing of foods and joining the glycemic index symbol program.

24. Berries—specifically, blueberries, blackberries, and raspberries—are among my favorite fruits. How do they affect my blood glucose level?

Some fruits have so little carbohydrate that they will have only a minor effect on blood glucose responses. Lucky for you, most berries have only 4 to 5 percent carbohydrate. Thus, a typical serving size (100 grams or 4 ounces) contains only 4 or 5 grams of carbohydrates. Furthermore, they are often very acidic, which means that if you eat them with another food (such as ice cream), the overall glycemic response will tend to be lower, because acids slow the emptying of food from the stomach. Next time you're tempted to have some ice cream, team it up with some of your favorite berries. You'll not only get the benefits of fruit, but also the calcium and other nutrients found in dairy foods.

25. Does cooking a food change its effect on my blood glucose? Would it be better to eat everything raw?

Whether or not cooking a food alters its effect on your blood glucose level depends on whether the food is based mainly on starch or mainly on sugars. Raw starch is not easily digested by human beings. In foods like potatoes, the raw starch is in a form that is almost totally resistant to digestion—eating raw potatoes is not only unpalatable but may result in gas and stomach cramps. That's why you don't see raw potatoes on menus!

In raw cereals, such as oats, the starch is present in a form that will be digested very slowly and result in a very low and gradual rise and fall in blood glucose. But in cooked cereals, the starch has gelatinized to a greater or lesser degree, which increases its rate of digestion and impact on blood glucose levels. The more severe the heating process, the higher the glycemic impact. In puffed and extruded snack products, the high temperatures and pressures bring about complete gelatinization of starch, leading to rapid digestion and absorption and a rapid rise in blood glucose. In contrast, the starch in cookies, for instance, is relatively ungelatinized and the glycemic impact is intermediate.

Cooling (refrigerating) cooked starch will further affect its structure and digestibility. Cooked potatoes and rice, when eaten cold, have a lower GI than when eaten freshly cooked. Even when the cooled product is reheated, the GI seems to remain lower than that of the freshly cooked product.

In foods such as fruit, the carbohydrate is present mainly in the form of sugars—glucose, fructose, and/or **sucrose**. Cooking will soften the cell walls of the fruit, but on the whole this won't make too much difference to the GI value. When we stop to think about it, the actual process of digestion in the stomach is equivalent to an "acid bath." The integrity of the cell walls will be destroyed in the stomach anyway.

So the answer to your question is no, it's not better to eat everything raw. Even from a vitamin point of view some studies have found that nutrient absorption is better from the cooked product than the raw food.

ALL ABOUT STARCH GELATINIZATION

Starch in raw food is contained in hard compact granules. During cooking, water and heat expand the starch granules to different degrees. Some granules actually burst and free the individual starch molecules. If most of the starch granules have swollen and burst during cooking, the starch is said to be fully gelatinized.

Swollen and free starch molecules are very rapidly digested in our intestine, because the digestive enzymes have a greater surface area to attack. The rapid digestion results in a rapid rise in blood glucose levels (remember that starch is a string of glucose molecules). A food containing fully gelatinized starch will therefore have a very high glycemic index. In the processing of cereal grains to make cold cereals like Corn Pops, Corn Flakes, and Rice Puffs, almost complete gelatinization of the starch is achieved, and the very slowly digested form of a whole cereal grain is converted to a very quickly digested form.

26. Does the carbohydrate content noted on a food's nutrition label have any relationship to its blood glucose–raising capacity?

Yes, but only to some extent. We can make a few generalizations. If the food has less than 5 grams of carbohydrate per serving, then it won't have a marked effect on your blood glucose levels. If it has 10 or more grams per serving, then it's likely to have a substantial effect, depending on the food's GI value. But, unfortunately, the carbohydrate content on the food label gives you no clue to its GI value.

What the label can tell you is whether the food is high or low in carbohydrate per serving. If it's high (e.g., above 10 grams per serving), then that tells us that it's a major source of carbohydrate in our diet, which makes the GI value more relevant. A food that is both high in carbohydrate and has a high GI value (e.g., bread) could be contributing to high blood glucose readings.

Studies tell us that diets based on frequent consumption of high GI value carbohydrates will put us at greatest risk of developing type 2 diabetes, heart disease, and some forms of cancer. It's not the amount of carbohydrate that matters as much as the source of the carbohydrate. High carbohydrate diets from only high glycemic index sources spell trouble, especially for people with insulin resistance, which is one of the underlying causes of type 2 diabetes.

27. What if I can't find a particular food in the glycemic index lists? I can't find tuna, eggs, chicken, avocado, kamut, jerusalem artichoke, jicama, macadamia nuts, spelt, textured vegetable protein, or triticale. Can I use the value given for a similar food?

Although there are now hundreds of foods tested for their effects on blood glucose levels, there are some foods that will never have an actual GI value. These include the protein foods that have no or little carbohydrate—tuna, eggs, chicken, and all manner of meat and fish and their substitutes, such as textured vegetable protein (TVP). Some plant foods, such as avocado, broccoli, and cucumber—all the salad vegetables, in fact—have negligible amounts of carbohydrate. Similarly, most nuts contain insignificant amounts of carbohydrate. Essentially, you can think of these foods as having a glycemic effect of zero—they won't markedly affect your blood glucose values. But some of the less commonly consumed carbohydrate foods, such as quinoa and triticale, still need to be tested.

Kamut is an ancient relative of durum wheat, and probably has a similar GI value.

Jerusalem artichoke, or sun choke (Helianthus tuberosus), is not related to the globe artichoke, the popular thistle grown in California. It has nothing to do with the city of Jerusalem (the name comes from the Italian word "girasola"). And, contrary to what you might read on some Internet sites and elsewhere, it has no "insulin." It contains something that is spelled similarly, *inulin*, which is an unavailable carbohydrate.

Jicama hasn't been tested yet and there are no plans to test it. It has only 4 percent available carbohydrate, so it is a **free food** in terms of the glycemic index.

Macadamia nuts have little available carbohydrate. They are about three-fourths fat and 8 percent protein, and 14 percent carbohydrate, of which 9 percent is fiber. In fact, their rich fat content gave rise to the common name of candle nuts in their country of origin, Australia. Australian Aborigines relished them. It is the only food native to Australia that has been commercially cultivated.

Spelt is an old-world form of wheat. The GI value of spelt wheat bread is 54, which is significantly lower than all the regular breads on the market. In fact, we suspect that most wild varieties of anything have a lower GI value than current cultivated varieties.

Textured vegetable protein (also known as TVP) is pure protein. It's made by spinning the gluten protein extracted from wheat flour into a texture that resembles meat. Any form of protein has relatively small effects on blood glucose levels (see question 63).

Triticale is a hybrid grain—a cross between a modern variety of wheat and rye. It hasn't been tested yet, but we suspect that triticale flour will be no different from wheat and rye in terms of glycemic index—that is, it will have a major effect on blood glucose levels.

Winter squashes: these haven't been tested for their GI values. The closest food is pumpkin. It was tested in South Africa, and so may be a different variety from what's available in North America. The GI value is 75. That it was this high is surprising and needs to be confirmed. Pumpkins are not a high source of carbohydrate anyway. Their orange color tells us that they are high in **carotenoids**—potent anti-oxidants—and that's a good reason to eat them in abundance.

28. There are many products on the market that have not been tested for their GI values. Is there some way I can estimate a food's glycemic effect by looking at the ingredients or the nutrition panel?

The ingredient list and "Nutrition Facts" panel will tell you the carbohydrate content, but it does not normally indicate the glycemic index. If it contains at least 10 grams per serving, you can be sure it will have at least some effect on your blood glucose concentration, but there is no way of telling whether it will be a little or a lot.

Furthermore, you can't readily estimate the GI value by looking at the ingredients or the nutrient composition, because so many factors have a bearing on it. By far, the most important factor is the final state of the starch, which depends on a whole array of factors: the amount of water in the food, the cooking time, the temperature and pressure during cooking, and the amount of sugar. The higher the sugar, the less the starch gelatinizes. The amount of viscous fiber, the acidity, and the concentration of sugars all affect the rate of digestion as well. Thus, foods high in things like psyllium and oat bran (both viscous fibers) may have a low glycemic index. More acidic fruits tend to have a lower GI value. More concentrated solutions of sugar also have lower GI values, because they are emptied more slowly from the stomach.

Although you can't guess the GI value of foods, there are some generalizations we can make about the glycemic index of different food categories. Legumes, for example, have some of the lowest GI values. Most pasta and noodle products tend to be low-GI foods, a fact that seems to surprise most folks. Most fresh fruits have a low GI value, but there are some important exceptions—for example, watermelon and cantalope have high GI values. Carbohydrate-rich dairy foods such as milk, yogurt, ice cream, and custard have low GI values. In contrast, most bread, bakery products, and cereals eaten in the United States have high GI values, but those which are less processed, and in which the grain is eaten in close to an intact physical form, will have lower GI values. Most types of rice are notable exceptions to this general rule (parboiled rice, however, has low GI values). It's also worth remembering that protein-rich foods, such as cheese, meat, fish, eggs, poultry, and green veggies don't have measurable GI values, because they contain little if any carbohydrate.

29. What is the glycemic load?

The glycemic load builds on our knowledge of the glycemic index. While the glycemic index measures the quality of the carbohydrate in different foods, the glycemic load reflects both the *quality* and the *quantity* of the carbohydrate in a typical serving.

The glycemic index compares the effect on our blood glucose of equal quantities of carbohydrates in different foods. What we mean by the quality of the carbohydrates here is their blood sugar–raising ability. A food with a high GI value contains carbs that are digested and absorbed more quickly than those in a food with a low glycemic index. However, the glycemic index doesn't tell you how many carbohydrates are in a serving of a particular food.

You need to know both the quality of the carbohydrates you eat and their quantity to understand a food's effect on your blood glucose level. That's where the glycemic load comes in.

Researchers at Harvard University introduced the concept of the glycemic load in 1997 to quantify the overall glycemic effect of a portion of food. However, only a few glycemic load values were calculated, and it was not possible to put it into practice until recently.

A team of researchers at the University of Sydney—including two of us, Jennie and Kaye—recently calculated the glycemic loads for all 750 foods for which we know the GI values. In the tables at the back of this book, we've listed the glycemic load of typical servings of hundreds of common foods, along with their GI value and carbohydrate content. Those figures and updates are also available on two Web sites: www.glycemicindex.com and www.mendosa.com/gilists.htm.

30. How do I calculate the glycemic load of a food?

Only the glycemic load can give us an estimate of the overall glycemic impact of a typical serving of food. It does this by multiplying the glycemic index of the food (expressed as a percentage) by the available carbohydrate in that serving.

Glycemic load = [grams of available carbohydrate per serving × GI] ÷ 100

Let's take a couple of examples:

Apples have a GI value of 38, and a medium-sized apple (4 ounces) contains about 15 grams of carbohydrate. The GL value for a medium apple is [15 × 38] ÷ 100 = 6.

Some varieties of potatoes have a GI value of 90, and an average serving of 5 ounces contains about 20 grams carbohydrate. Their GL value is [20 × 90] ÷ 100 = 18.

So a typical serving of potatoes can be expected to have three times the glycemic effect of an apple.

Sometimes the results are surprising. Watermelon, for example, has a rather high glycemic index, 72. A large serving of 8 ounces has only 12 grams of available carbohydrate. So watermelon's glycemic load is [12 × 72] ÷ 100 = 8.

The glycemic load of a food is the product of its glycemic index and its carbohydrate content. So both factors have a role in determining it. Which is more important? Statistical analysis shows that the carbohydrate content by itself explains 68 percent of the variation in glycemic load values among foods, while the GI value explains about half. So, while carbohydrate is clearly a greater contributor, they are both important!

What the glycemic load tells us is that it's helpful to limit those foods that have both a high GI value and high carbohydrate content (e.g., potatoes, breakfast cereals, breads, rice, and other cereal products).

31. In blood glucose terms, how do I compare a small banana with a large apple, or a plate of pasta with a serving of rice?

To predict and compare the overall blood glucose response to foods, we must calculate the glycemic load. To do this we need to know both the GI value and the available carbohydrate content of the food (carbohydrates minus fiber). Next, calculate the glycemic load of each portion:

Glycemic load = [grams of available carbohydrate per serving × GI] ÷ 100

Let's do an example. A small banana contains 21 grams of available carbohydrate per serving and has a GI value of 52.

GL = [21 × 52] ÷ 100 = 10.9

A large apple contains 27 grams of available carbohydrate per serving and has a GI value of 38.

GL = [27 × 38] ÷ 100 = 10.3

So the small banana has much the same effect as a large apple. Take your pick! Now, let's take the average plate of pasta and compare with the serving of rice. A plate of spaghetti weighs 180 grams and contains about 48 grams of carbohydrate. Its GI value is about 40.

GL = [48 × 40] ÷ 100 = 19.2

A typical serving of Jasmine rice weighs 150 grams and contains about 42 grams of carbohydrate. Its GI value is 109.

$$GL = [42 \times 109] \div 100 = 45.8$$

Comparing 46 with 19, suggests that the serving of rice will have more than twice the impact of the plate of pasta.★ That's a big difference!

★In a healthy individual, the glycemic response may not be twice as high because he or she is able to secrete more insulin in response to the rapidly rising blood glucose level. The insulin demand, however, will be approximately two times higher.

32. To calculate the glycemic load, should I use total carbohydrate or available carbohydrate?

It's important when we calculate the glycemic load that we base it only on the *available* carbohydrate in a food (see question 19). This means, if we are using food composition figures from the United States, we need to first work out the available carbohydrate by subtracting fiber from the total carbohydrate. You may recall from question 19 that fiber is *unavailable carbohydrate*, that is, not available for digestion. All of our glycemic load calculations are based on the available carbohydrate content of the foods tested.

Previously, the glycemic loads for only a very few foods had been calculated. The book *Eat, Drink, and Be Healthy*, by Walter C. Willett (Simon & Schuster, 2001), listed the glycemic loads for 34 foods. Unfortunately, those GL calculations are not comparable to those published elsewhere. All of them are based on setting bread as equal to 100 on the glycemic index scale. Furthermore, the calculations were based on total (rather than available) carbohydrate, so they overestimate the true glycemic load. Our GL calculations use the more common index, where glucose (rather than bread) is set to equal 100.

33. What do you consider to be a high glycemic load and a low glycemic load? In other words, what cutoffs can be used to classify foods as high, intermediate, or low glycemic load (GL)?

At this stage we suggest you use a cutoff of 20 or above for high-GL values and 10 or below for low-GL values. That means that foods with GL values between 11 and 19 are in the intermediate range.

It makes sense to use these values for the time being, while further research is being conducted. When we set cutoffs for high, medium, and low-GI values back in 1996, we based the values on pragmatic considerations. Looking at the range of values and the variety of foods, these cutoffs seemed practical from a dietetic perspective and could be used to help people reduce the GI values of their diets. It's too early to tell what glycemic load cutoffs will be useful in practice. That's because total glycemic load should be related to energy intake. The higher our energy requirements, the higher our carbohydrate intake and, naturally, the higher the glycemic load (since it is a measure of carbohydrate quantity times glycemic index).

LOW GL . . . OR HIGH?

For average-sized servings of individual foods, we suggest the following criteria to judge whether the food has a high or low glycemic load.

High GL = 20 or above
Intermediate GL = 11–19
Low GL = 10 or below

34. Wouldn't it be better to consider a food's glycemic load instead of its glycemic index value when comparing foods? In other words, what's more important—a food's GI value or its GL value?

Both a food's GI value and its GL value are important. Some people have argued that glycemic load is an advance on GI values, because it provides an estimate of both quantity and quality of carbohydrate (GI value gives us just quality) in a diet. However, the risk of disease is predicted by both the glycemic index as well as the glycemic load. The use of the glycemic load corroborates the findings of the glycemic index, suggesting that the more frequent the consumption of high-carbohydrate, high-GI value foods, the more adverse the health outcome. The data does not suggest that a lower carbohydrate intake is protective.

Use common sense when considering the glycemic load of a food. Low-carbohydrate foods will always have a low GL value, but we don't recommend low-carbohydrate diets. Carbohydrate content alone shows absolutely no relationship to disease risk. In the Harvard studies (see question 29), the low risk of disease associated with the lowest glycemic load was driven by the consumption of foods with a low GI, not by foods with a low carbohydrate content. So our message here is don't aim for foods that have a low carbohydrate content and a lot of fat, especially saturated fat (e.g., cream, bacon, salami). Diets based on these foods might have a low glycemic load, but they could also put you at risk of developing heart disease.

Use the GI value to compare foods of similar nature (bread with bread, breakfast cereal with breakfast cereal).

Consider the glycemic load when a food has a high GI value but low carbohydrate content per normal serving. People say that's why the glycemic load is superior to GI value, but there are remarkably few foods in this category (watermelon, cantaloupe, pumpkin, rutabaga, broad beans). New research shows carrots have neither a high GI nor high GL (see question 80).

Some people have also asked us which foods have low GI values but high GL values. In our lists, these foods include: cakes, cookies, some chocolate candy, and some fruit juice drinks. These are foods we should limit for a whole variety of reasons, besides their high GL values.

35. Is the glycemic load as scientific and *objective* as the glycemic index?

Yes, glycemic load and glycemic index are both objective measures, but glycemic load still needs further research to prove its worth. We need proof that portions of different foods that have the same glycemic load do indeed produce similar blood glucose responses. We need evidence that the concept predicts blood glucose levels when we eat two or even three servings in one sitting. We need to know if it is predictive in the context of a "mixed meal" based on several different foods. Lastly, the glycemic load concept needs to be compared with the measurement of simple carbohydrate as far as determining insulin requirements, especially for insulin pump users. Research in these areas is being pursued at present.

There is one subjective element to the glycemic load, and that is the portion or serving sizes for which there are no international standards. Different individuals, of course, eat different amounts. And each of us doesn't always eat the same amount. So the size of the portion or serving on which the glycemic load of a food is based can make a considerable difference.

36. Is there evidence that a healthy individual with no indications or risk factors suggesting susceptibility to diabetes will benefit from a low-GI diet?

There is certainly good scientific evidence suggesting you will live a healthier life. In the Nurses Health Study, a large-scale epidemiological study carried out by the Harvard School of Public Health, women who were naturally eating a low-GI diet were half as likely to have a heart attack. Both men and women were less likely to develop type 2 diabetes.

In other studies, low-GI diets were associated with improvements in indicators for heart disease risk. These included lower levels of LDL-cholesterol and triglycerides, lower levels of inflammatory markers, and higher levels of the good HDL-cholesterol. These effects of low-GI diets were not simply because low-GI diets might be higher in fiber. In fact, a diet that was both low in GI values *and* high in fiber combined the best of both worlds, and was associated with the lowest risk of all.

In a small number of studies, low-GI diets resulted in greater weight loss compared with conventional high-carbohydrate diets. There is also some evidence that low-GI diets reduce the risk of breast cancer in women, colon cancer in men, and pancreatic cancer in both men and women. However, further studies are needed before we can be confident that the findings are "cause and effect," and not simply coincidental.

You might be wondering why the GI values of foods would have such far-reaching effects. The most likely reason is the effect on blood glucose and insulin levels. Insulin is a hormone with a whole multitude of effects. If high-GI value foods create an excessive demand for insulin, it is possible that the cells that produce insulin may become "exhausted," thereby triggering diabetes. High levels of glucose in the bloodstream after meals could also be responsible for a whole host of undesirable effects that lead, over the longer term, to weight gain and heart disease.

What Makes My Blood Glucose Go Up?

Food Factors That Increase My Blood Glucose Levels

37. What are the worst foods for raising blood glucose levels?

Of those foods that we eat regularly, two stand out as having very high glycemic potential.

Most extreme are potatoes. Not only do they usually have a high glycemic index, they have a high carbohydrate content, and some people eat them in enormous quantities. This combination makes them a major contributor to high blood glucose levels. Foremost among potatoes is the variety, originally developed by the brilliant horticulturalist Luther Burbank (1849–1926), known as the Russet Burbank. Ideally suited for growing in Idaho and baking in the oven, it is *less than* ideal for your blood glucose.

While a baked Russet Burbank potato won't raise your blood glucose as much as the same amount of glucose, it will raise it quite a bit more than sucrose, or table sugar. And it's not just baked potatoes that can do you in, at least in terms of your blood glucose. Even mashed potatoes and french fries have higher blood glucose-raising abilities than table sugar.

Besides potatoes, the other common food that raises our blood glucose markedly is wheat flour. Though you may think that you don't eat much of it, it is a common ingredient in bread, crackers, most breakfast cereals, and bagels. All of these foods are among the highest in raising blood glucose.

Sugary and some starchy foods can also be the villains if you eat exceptionally large quantities. A glass of soft drink is fine, but a "big gulp" or quart isn't. A few jelly beans are okay, but not the bag. A small bowl of pasta is not going to raise your blood glucose level too far, but a double serving will. So be sensible and exercise moderation in your portion sizes. Be especially wary of those "value-for-money" deals where you get a huge serving at marginally increased cost—unless, of course, you plan to share it with a friend.

38. Why do small new potatoes affect blood glucose levels less than bigger potatoes?

Potatoes have been the subject of dozens of studies. On the whole, they have a very marked effect on blood glucose, similar to that of pure glucose, on a gram-for-gram of carbohydrate basis. In studies, new potatoes (also known as chats or cocktail potatoes) produced a moderate glycemic effect, although some were better than others. We suspect the smaller they are, the lower their effect on blood sugar. However, it's too early to conclude that all new potatoes will have lower GI values than more mature spuds.

Interestingly, in one study of several potato varieties, the investigators noticed a correlation between the size of the tuber and its GI value—the bigger the potato, the higher the GI value. Hence new potatoes may indeed have lower GI values simply because of their smaller size. But why should size matter? Food chemists have noted that as a potato matures, the starch molecule becomes more and more branched. Hence, a new potato containing starch with less branching may behave differently during the cooking process. Scientists know that long unbranched starch chains have a habit of lining up in rows, attracting each other with very strong bonds. In this way, the starch in new potatoes may be more resistant to enzymic digestion. More studies are clearly needed.

At present, we don't know whether some of these differences among potato varieties are due to errors in estimating their true carbohydrate content. Potatoes can vary from as little as 11 percent to up to 20 percent carbohydrate, but in many studies, the carbohydrate content has not been determined directly on the product being tested—the value was simply taken from food composition tables. If the amount of carbohydrate per 100 grams has been overestimated, then the weight of a 50 gram carbohydrate portion will be lower, and the resulting GI value will be lower than it should be.

Some people have also wondered why potatoes are almost unique among the starchy vegetables in producing such high glycemic responses. It's possible that their high GI value results from thousands of years of careful plant selection to pick the biggest yielding plants—those that produce the biggest and best potatoes. Bigger potatoes may mean greater **amylopectin** branching and, therefore, higher GI value. Alternatively, potatoes that are more palatable may have higher degrees of gelatinization when cooked, which we know correlates with the glycemic index. What this means is that some varieties of "wild" or "gourmet" potatoes, such as fingerlings or pink fir apple, may have lower GI values.

THE GI VALUES OF POTATOES

Potatoes	Glycemic index	Glycemic load
Baked without fat	85	26
Boiled	88	16
Mashed	92	18
Instant mashed	85	17
French fries	75	22
Canned	63	11
Chips	57	10
Canadian baked (Russet)	56	10
Canadian baked (Ontario)	58	10

39. Do I have to avoid eating potatoes and bread because they have high GI values?

It depends. If you are overly fond of potatoes and bread, you'd better steer clear of them for your own sake. If it's all or nothing, then nothing is better for you than large servings of either bread or potatoes.

Most of us, however, can control our potato or bread intakes. If that's your style, you might find that a small portion is better than total withdrawal.

It can also help if you choose those potatoes and flour products that raise your blood glucose less than typical for these foods. For example, try new potatoes, which are simply young potatoes of any variety and, as explained in the previous question, are shown to have less effect on your blood glucose level. Some of the new, small "gourmet" potato varieties, such as Yukon Gold, are also likely to contain slowly digested starch, but we need to await further testing before we can be sure. In the meantime, you might like to experiment a bit on yourself.

When it comes to breads, your best choices are sourdough, stone-ground, pumpernickel, and any similar bread where you can see the intact kernels of grain with the naked eye. They will raise blood glucose levels less than typical white or whole wheat bread.

It all comes down to quantity and quality. The worse the quality—that is the higher a food's GI value—the less of it that you can safely eat without it severely affecting your blood glucose.

40. Does bread made from sprouted grains have less blood glucose-raising potential than bread made from flour?

We don't yet know the answer to this one. Bread made from sprouted grains might well have a lower blood glucose-raising ability than bread made from normal flour. Why's that? When grains begin to sprout, carbohydrates stored in the grain are used as the fuel source for the new shoot. Chances are that the more readily available carbohydrates stored in the wheat grain will be used up first, thereby reducing the amount in the final product. Furthermore, if the *whole kernel* form of the wheat grain is retained in the finished product, it will have the desired effect of lowering the blood glucose level. Physically limiting access of digestive enzymes to the starchy endosperm helps to reduce the rate of starch digestion.

41. Rice appears to vary in its blood glucose-raising ability. Is there a way I can tell the difference?

You can use the eating quality or texture of the rice as a guide to its likely effect on blood glucose. The stickier the rice, the higher the glycemic potency. The rice commonly served in Chinese restaurants is sticky rice, which often has a relatively high blood glucose-raising ability. Jasmine rice, often served in Thai restaurants, is also extremely potent, as is Arborio, the rice traditionally used to make risotto. Rice varieties in which the cooked grains are clearly separated from each other and "drier" in texture are more slowly digested and therefore less potent. The best example is Basmati rice, which is often served in Indian restaurants and with curries. You can easily pick out a single grain of Basmasti rice.

The reason that rices vary so much in their blood glucose-raising abilities is that they vary in proportions of two types of starches—amylopectin and **amylose**. Amylopectin is the most readily digestible form of starch, as opposed to amylose, which is harder to digest. This is because amylose is a straight-chain molecule that has tight bonding between the strands, while amylopectin is highly branched, making the structure more open to water absorption.

If you are fond of sushi, then you'll be pleased to hear that it appears to have a low blood glucose-raising potential. This may be because sushi is made with vinegar and nori (seaweed) in addition to rice. The vinegar slows down stomach emptying and therefore the rate of digestion. The soluble viscous fiber in the seaweed helps lower the glycemic response. Sashimi (raw fish) won't raise blood glucose levels at all because there's no carbohydrate to speak of.

You can't use the size of the rice grain to judge a rice's glycemic potency, as long or short-grain rices are available in both high-GI and low-GI varieties. Similarly, parboiled (converted) rices can be slowly or rapidly digested, depending on the variety. In North America most converted rices have a low GI value. Uncle Ben's converted rice, for example, has a GI value of only 50.

These guidelines are only rough guides, however, not guarantees. If you'd like to know more about your favorite rice, write to the manufacturer and ask them to have it tested for its GI value by a well-established testing laboratory.

42. Does brown rice have a lower effect on blood glucose levels than white rice?

Surprisingly, brown rice can have a high glycemic potency, despite its higher fiber content. But we know little about brown rice because very few tests have been performed.

Many people are surprised to hear that a whole-grain food like brown rice can have such a high GI value. Under the microscope, a rice grain, whether brown or white, can be seen to have thousands of cracks and fissures. This gives easy access for water absorption during cooking. Heat and water together allow almost complete gelatinization of the starch to take place in a relatively short period of time. In comparison, a whole-wheat grain has no cracks and takes much longer to cook.

43. How is it that some foods can have GI values of over 100?

While pure glucose is theoretically the food with the highest blood glucose-raising ability (i.e., 100), there are some substances that empty from the stomach faster than glucose, and are very quickly digested and absorbed. One of these is **maltose**, a double sugar containing two glucose molecules. Another is corn syrup solids, a common sweetener based on short-chain glucose polymers ("short strings" of glucose). When dissolved in water, both maltose and corn syrup solids exert less **osmotic pressure**, or pull, on the lining of the small intestine. This makes them more easily absorbed and results in GI values over 100.

Dried dates and tofu frozen desert have recorded GI values greater than 100. More recently, scientists tested several other varieties of dates and found they had a relatively low GI value (in the range 30 to 50). In retrospect, the first value obtained was probably incorrect. If the carbohydrate content is not reliable, this can lead to errors in GI value estimation. The errors can be magnified with foods that lose water during storage, such as dried fruits.

It's also possible that all the carbohydrate in the tofu frozen dessert comes from a mixture of **dextrose** and **maltodextrin**s (see the discussion of dextrose and maltodextrins in question 44).

In our experience, it's best not to rely too heavily on the GI value of a food that has been tested only once and gives a surprisingly high or low value. In the searchable glycemic index database online (www.glycemicindex.com), you can easily see how many times a food has been tested. A good percentage of foods have been tested at least twice.

44. I am currently using a protein bar that contains maltodextrin. I've noticed that many sports drinks list both maltodextrins and dextrose. What's the difference between the two? Is one better than the other?

Maltodextrins are short-chain glucose polymers that are readily digested. They are made by partial breakdown of starch. We can think of starch as a long strand of pearls where each pearl is a glucose molecule. If you chopped the strand into individual pearls, you'd have pure glucose. Glucose also goes by the name of "dextrose" and is very sweet.

If we chopped the long strand of pearls into several short pieces, however, we would have a mixture of short-chain glucose polymers, or "maltodextrins." Usually there are a mixture of polymers present, some with two, three, or four glucose residues per chain, and others with five or six. These don't taste sweet, but they are readily digested and absorbed—more so than either pure starch or pure glucose. That's because starch needs to be highly gelatinized to be digested fast, while pure glucose exerts such a high osmotic pressure★ in the stomach that it slows down stomach emptying.

That's why sports drinks contain a mixture of both maltodextrins and dextrose. The mixture exerts the same osmotic pressure as blood, so the solution is emptied

★Osmotic pressure is the force exerted by molecules as they bump and bounce off cell walls and membranes. At the same concentration, a solution of small molecules exerts a greater pressure than a solution of large molecules. Hence a 10-percent glucose solution exerts more osmotic pressure than a 10-percent solution of maltodextrins.

quickly. Sports drink manufacturers want fast absorption to meet the demand for energy, but if they used pure glucose it would not only be sickly sweet, it would also be absorbed less quickly.

45. Why are people with diabetes now allowed to eat sugar?

Sugar has had a bad rap, some of it deserved, most of it not. It is true that sugar has absolutely no nutritional value. It has calories and sweetness but no micronutrients. But this can be said about pure starch, protein, fat, and alcohol. And we consume all of these without a second thought!

But in moderation neither calories nor sweetness is such a bad thing. We need calories to live, and we have a natural craving for sweetness. A little sugar won't hurt most of us. What *does* hurt is the attitude of well-meaning people. A reader with **type 1 diabetes** told us the following story:

> I once went to a dinner party given by a very high-ranking professional, where everyone was served dessert except for me. But the host never bothered to ask whether or not I could have dessert—he just made the assumption that because I had diabetes, I couldn't have anything with sugar. I was, frankly, appalled at this behavior.

If you find yourself in a similar situation, be assertive and say, "Hey, didn't you know the rules have changed? Everyone, including those with diabetes, can enjoy dessert." It makes great dinner table conversation!

Some of us, however, may be "addicted" to sugar. We say we can't get enough of it. This is the argument behind the best-selling book, *Sugar Blues* by William F. Dufty, originally published in 1975 and still in print. Twenty-five years later, *Sugar Blues* inspired the popular diet book, *Sugar Busters!*

But there isn't any real evidence that sugar is "addictive" in the strict sense of the word. That is, we don't experience dramatic symptoms of withdrawal when it's unavailable. Sugar in moderation won't even have a huge effect on your blood glucose.

In fact, if you ate the same amount of a wheat cereal that came with sugar added it would have much the same effect on your blood glucose as wheat cereal without added sugar. Sugar has a glycemic index of about 65, while whole wheat cereal (like Shredded Wheat) is 75.

In May 1994, the American Diabetes Association (ADA) stopped recommending that people with diabetes avoid sugar. The ADA's revised guidelines, originally published in the organization's professional journal, *Diabetes Care*, and subsequently in its position statement, "Nutrition Recommendations and Principles for People with Diabetes Mellitus," say essentially that previous guidelines concerning sugar were mistaken:

> "For most of this century, the most widely held belief about the nutritional treatment of diabetes has been that simple sugars should be avoided and replaced with starches. This belief appears to be based on the assumption that sugars are more rapidly digested and absorbed than are starches and thereby aggravate hyperglycemia to a greater degree. There is, however, very little scientific evidence that supports this assumption."

When people tell you that someone who has diabetes can't eat anything with sugar in it, you know they are a bit out of date. Table sugar (sucrose), and other sweeteners like honey, molasses, maple syrup, and cane syrup are okay if eaten in moderation.

46. From the perspective of blood glucose, is honey better than sugar?

Up until recently, we would have said honey is no different from sugar. After all, honey doesn't contribute much in the way of micronutrients, and we thought it had a similar effect on blood glucose as table sugar. In fact, one commercial honey from Canada was found to have a greater effect than sugar itself.

But more recent evidence suggests that some forms of honey have only a minor effect on blood glucose. These are the pure floral honeys—red gum, yellow box, ironbark, and others—that have been produced by allowing the bees access to only some types of gum trees. It's possible that all pure floral honeys have only modest glycemic effects, but it's too early to say. Romanian locust honey appears to have the lowest effect of all the honeys. Still, most commercial varieties have the same or greater effect as table sugar.

Why would one honey be different from another? Well, most commercial honeys are made from a mixture of honeys, derived from different hives and floral sources. To maintain a consistent flavor, some of the more pungent characteristics are removed. We suspect that the components that are removed are physiologically active and work to slow down absorption. For example, Australian floral honeys might contain **alpha–glucosidase inhibitors** that bees have extracted from the flowers of the gums.

We know that these potent inhibitors exist in many plants and, indeed, some diabetic medications (e.g., Acarbose) are based on pure forms of these inhibitors.

47. Do you know of any comparisons between molasses and ordinary white table sugar? What about cane sugar?

We don't know the answer to that one because testing has not been carried out. It's possible that molasses, the rather bitter tasting sweet syrup left at the end of the refining process, might have lower blood glucose-raising ability than table sugar. Molasses comes in colors ranging from dark brown to gold. We suspect that there may be natural components present which could possibly reduce the rate of digestion and absorption. The darker the molasses, the better.

Some of the gourmet varieties of cane sugar such as Sucanat, Turbinado, and Sugar in the Raw have varying degrees of color and crystal size, and there may be a difference in their rate of digestion and absorption (see question 44). There are probably more minerals and even some other nutrients in them, that may influence enzyme activity or stomach emptying.

48. How much sugar is okay?

Our understanding of sugar's overall effect on health has changed considerably over the last ten to fifteen years. The consensus from a recent World Health Organization report on the role of sugar in the diet is that "a moderate intake of sugar-rich foods can provide for a palatable and nutritious diet." So what's moderate?

Most health authorities would consider sixty grams (about two ounces) of refined sugar a moderate and acceptable daily amount of sugar for most individuals. That's about ten percent of total energy intake. The trouble is that average consumption in the United States is close to triple that! The U.S. Department of Agriculture says that in 1996, Americans consumed an average of 153 pounds of caloric sweeteners per year, a 20-percent increase in ten years. This works out to more than 190 grams or six ounces per person per day, or 16 percent of total energy intake.

Of course, many people are consuming even more than the average. Some of them, such as heavy laborers and endurance athletes, may need this source of readily available energy. However, most Americans lead inactive lives and therefore need to cut down their sugar intake to reach sixty grams per day. But there's no need to go to extremes and completely avoid it.

At moderate levels of intake, sugar is deemed to have no effect on disease risk, apart from tooth decay. In relation to obesity, most studies in adults and children have shown that those whose diets are relatively high in sugar or sugar-containing foods are no heavier than their peers. In some countries, the dramatic rise in obesity has been accompanied by a decline in sugar consumption. In addition, sugar shows a reciprocal relationship with intake of saturated fat. Those who eat sugar in moderation have lower intakes of saturated fats.

A moderate intake of added caloric sweeteners is sixty grams per day. That's equivalent to ten teaspoons of sugar or one-and-a-half cans of soft drink. The box below shows the sugar content of other types of sweets.

ADDED CALORIC SWEETENER CONTENT OF VARIOUS FOODS (IN GRAMS)

1 teaspoon of sugar	6
1 tablespoon of jam	11
1 piece of hard candy	5
5 squares of chocolate	20
1 chocolate bar (average)	35
12-ounce can of soft drink	40
1 cream-filled cookie	5
1 piece of chocolate cake	11
1 cinnamon and sugar doughnut	7

49. Should I avoid high-fructose corn syrup?

The value of including fructose in the diet has been a source of controversy in the nutrition world for several years. Fructose does not raise blood glucose levels as much as sucrose (table sugar), but some studies show it to have a deleterious effect on blood fats. Generally, these findings only apply when fructose is consumed in very large amounts, and there are many studies that show no deleterious effects of moderate amounts

High-fructose corn syrup is used by food manufacturers primarily as a sweetener. Although the fructose component may sound attractive due to its minor impact on blood glucose—pure fructose has a GI value of nineteen—most high-fructose corn syrup is about 50-percent fructose. The other 50 percent is glucose, making the predicted GI value no less than 60—around the same as regular sugar or sucrose. Purified fructose is a relatively expensive commodity that is less frequently used in food manufacture, so the practical benefit of fructose is somewhat limited. Nevertheless, the presence of fructose in honey and fruits is beneficial in lowering blood glucose levels.

A recent study showed that a small amount of fructose (about two teaspoons) consumed just before a high-carbohydrate meal reduced the overall glycemic effect of the meal. The mechanism may be related to the fact that fructose consumption inhibits the formation of new glucose by the liver. So a small priming amount of fructose gives the liver a "head start."

50. There are times when I crave something sweet. What should I have?

Many people experience times when they crave something sweet. Part of this stems from an instinctual liking for sweet foods—part of the hard wiring in our brains that tells us that a food that is sweet is a safe source of energy. Craving something sweet may also be a signal you are hungry. Trying to deny the instinct to eat something sweet can be a "no-win" situation. Perhaps the best strategy is to take care so that in satisfying your desire for something sweet, you don't overdo your fat intake. Sweet-fat combinations like cakes, chocolate, and cookies contain more energy as fat than they do as sugar!

What you choose depends on your tastes, but here's a list of ideas to get you started:

- Jam on low-GI toast
- Dried apples or apricots
- Dates
- A low-fat flavored milk
- Canned fruit cocktail
- A pure floral honey
- Low-fat ice cream
- Low-fat yogurt or pudding
- Fresh peaches
- Fresh berries of any form
- A dried fruit bar

If you just desire a sweet taste in your mouth, artificially sweetened products—like diet or low-calorie soft drinks or artificially sweetened candy—can fit the bill.

Alternatively, go ahead and have a hard candy, especially one that takes a long time to dissolve, such as barley sugar. Take one and get yourself busy with something to take your mind off eating. One hard candy supplies about four grams of sugar—not enough to have much effect on your blood glucose levels at all—and at only fifteen calories it's nothing to feel guilty about.

51. Is there a difference between "natural" sugars in foods and added sugars?

The sugars found naturally in fruits, vegetables, dairy products, and honey are no different chemically from the sugars we add to foods, so our body does not distinguish between them. Sucrose—the sugar that we put in our sugar bowl—is absolutely identical to the source of sweetness in fruit. It is a **disaccharide** composed of glucose and fructose. It is these sugars that give fruit and certain vegetables (such as carrots and peas) their sweetness. The mild sweetness of milk comes from another disaccharide, **lactose**, composed of glucose and galactose.

The rates of digestion and absorption of these different sugars are reflected in their GI values:

- ▶ Fructose   19
- ▶ Lactose   46
- ▶ Sucrose   68
- ▶ Glucose   100

We can see from this how the intermediate GI value of sucrose comes about, given the GI values of its component sugars: 50-percent fructose plus 50-percent glucose. Honey, another added sugar, is composed of varying proportions of glucose, fructose, and sucrose, and has an average GI value 55—it ranges from as low as 32 for a pure floral honey to a high of 87 for a nondescript blend. We say more about honey in question 46.

High-fructose corn syrup (sometimes labeled as corn syrup solids) is another added sugar which is widely used by manufacturers in the United States. These are glucose syrups made from hydrolyzed corn starch and have high blood glucose-raising ability. Non-diet soft drinks are the greatest source of sugars in the American diet, accounting for one-third of the average person's intake of sugars. Almost all of the added sugar in soft drinks is high-fructose corn syrup. You can read more about that in question 49.

GI values within groups of foods containing added or naturally occurring sugars vary greatly. The GI value of fruits varies from 22 for cherries to 72 for watermelon. Similarly, among foods containing refined sugar, some have a low GI and some a high one. The GI value of sweetened yogurt is only 33, while a Mars Bar has a GI value of 62 (lower than bread).

Some nutritionists argue that naturally occurring sugars are better because they come packaged with other vitamins and minerals often not associated with foods high in refined sugars. In some foods, such as fruit, this may be the case, but likewise, the addition of sugar to a nutritious food, such as yogurt, make it more palatable. Diet quality is, in fact, positively associated with sugar intake. Studies that have analyzed high and low-sugar diets clearly show them to contain similar amounts of micronutrients.

52. Are sweet potatoes a good substitute for regular potatoes, even though they are sweet? Are sweet potatoes and yams the same thing?

There is a big difference between a regular potato and a sweet potato, not only in appearance but also in glycemic potency. The flesh of regular potatoes is usually white or creamy yellow and occasionally gold in color, but sweet potatoes are usually orange or pink in color. This difference is due to the presence of natural color substances called *carotenoids*—the deeper the yellow color, the greater their concentration. Their shape differs too. While regular potatoes are usually irregularly shaped spheres, sweet potatoes are large, long root-shaped tubers. Beyond these easily visible differences, sweet potatoes will raise your blood glucose levels *significantly less* than potatoes. This makes them an excellent substitute.

Regular potatoes and sweet potatoes don't even belong to the same family. The potato is a tuber of a member of the nightshade family and was originally cultivated in South America. The sweet potato is the root of a member of the morning glory family and is also native to South America.

It's hard to confuse potatoes and sweet potatoes. In the United States we sometimes use the word *yam* to describe what is really a sweet potato simply because their shapes are similar. The so-called garnet and jewel "yams" are actually sweet potatoes. In fact, yams and sweet potatoes aren't even distantly related. A yam is the tuber of tropical vine belonging to the family called *Dioscorea*. True yams are still eaten by Australian Aboriginal people leading semi-traditional lifestyles in remote parts of Australia. Testing them has shown that they produce very low blood glucose responses. Cheeky yam, for example, has a glycemic index of only 34.

WHAT'S SO GOOD ABOUT CAROTENES?

Carotenes are the orange-yellow colored pigments in plants that our body can convert to vitamin A. Vitamin A keeps our skin healthy, helps in our resistance to infections, and helps us see in dim light—hence the adage that carrots are good for your eyesight. Beta-carotene, which is found in carrots, has the highest levels of vitamin A activity. Other orange and yellow fruits and vegetables, including pumpkin, peaches, cantalope, mango, and apricots, are also high in carotenes. Green and red vegetables, such as spinach, peppers, and broccoli, also contain carotenes, but their presence is masked by the green pigment chlorophyll.

53. Are rolled oats good for blood glucose levels? Does it matter which type?

What we call rolled oats or oatmeal in the United States goes by the name porridge in the United Kingdom and most of the rest of the English-speaking world. By whatever name, this common breakfast cereal is slowly digested and absorbed and won't have a marked effect on your blood glucose.

Traditional porridge has a medium GI value (around the 50 mark), which indicates a moderate blood glucose-raising potential. Instant oatmeal, however, has a greater ability to raise your blood glucose level (its GI is 66).

Because of their larger particle size, there's good reason to believe that steel-cut oats have less blood glucose-raising ability than regular rolled oats. Steel-cut oats are whole grain groats—the inner portion of the oat kernel—which have been cut into only two or three pieces. Rolled oats are flake oats that have been steamed, rolled, re-steamed, and toasted.

A simple guide to the glycemic potential of rolled oats is the time it takes to cook them—if they cook up nicely in one minute, chances are they'll have a fairly marked effect on your blood glucose. If they take fifteen minutes or more, they are likely to be less potent.

54. I have a habit of popping a 4-quart pot full of popcorn two or three times per week, and I eat all of it watching a movie. Is that a bad thing?

There are worse snacks than popcorn, but there are several aspects of this question that are troubling. The first is the sheer volume and energy content of food ingested—about half the average requirement for the whole day! The second is that the vast majority of the calories are in the form of trans fat or saturated fat—the worst thing for your heart and blood vessels. Third, you eat all that food while expending very little energy. A good recipe for weight gain, if that's your aim.

Popcorn is also a high-GI value food, and that amount will raise your blood glucose level substantially. Check your blood two hours after you start to nibble it and see how it affects you.

If you do eat popcorn, try to limit yourself by nibbling slowly and limiting the amount in the bowl to a few handfuls. Also make sure not to use any microwave-ready packages, because these are loaded with partially hydrogenated oil, also known as trans fat, the very worst fat. Pop your own and eat it with a little butter, which of course has saturated fat. But saturated fat is not as bad for you as partially hydrogenated oil.

THE VERY WORST FAT: TRANS FAT

Trans fat is found in vegetable shortenings, some margarines, crackers, cookies, and many other foods made with or fried in partially hydrogenated fats. The following information is from a 1995 report from the U.S. Department of Agriculture. Measurements indicate grams per serving.

Margarine (stick)
1.8–3.5

Vegetable shortening
1.4–4.2

Salad dressings (regular)
0.06–1.1

Margarine (tub, regular)
0.4–1.6

Pound cake
4.3

Vegetable oils
0.01–0.06

Microwave popcorn (regular)
2.2

Doughnuts
0.3–3.8

Vanilla wafers
1.3

Chocolate chip cookies
1.2–2.7

Snack crackers
1.8–2.5

French fries (fast food)
0.7–3.6

Chocolate candies
0.04–2.8

Snack chips
0–1.2

Ready-to-eat breakfast cereal
0.05–0.5

White bread
0.06–0.7

B.

Non-Food Factors That Increase Blood Glucose Levels

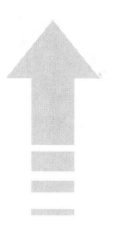

55. Did gaining weight as I got older give me the high blood glucose levels I have now?

Yes, you can bet on that. As you gain weight, the cells of your body become resistant, or "blind," to the insulin secreted by your pancreas into your bloodstream. Why? The more fat you have, especially fat around the middle, the more the body tries to use it as a source of fuel. When glucose starts streaming into the blood subsequent to a meal, it has to compete with the fat already in the "engine room." To displace the fat as the fuel source, more insulin must be manufactured to channel glucose into the cells and keep blood glucose levels under control. In a nutshell, that's what we mean by insulin resistance. You'll recall from question 1 that the body tries to keep blood glucose levels within a fairly narrow range, not too high, not too low.

Some of us are born with an unlimited capacity to make extra insulin day after day, year after year. But others reach a point where the effort involved is overwhelming and the insulin-producing cells go on strike—they are exhausted. Then, blood glucose levels start to climb higher and higher after each meal.

It's clear when you look around at your family and friends that not every large person has diabetes. While more than 60 percent of Americans are overweight, only about 6 percent have diabetes. Diabetes is more common in some ethnic groups than in others, probably for genetic reasons. The most affected group is Native Americans, while people of Asian, African-American, and Hispanic origins are also at higher risk. Even a little excess weight around the waistline puts people at greater risk.

Yet not everyone with type 2 diabetes is carrying extra pounds. Some people with type 2 diabetes are extraordinarily lean. For one reason or another, the insulin-producing cells have gone out on strike.

You can fight back against insulin resistance directly with exercise, which makes your body's cells more receptive to insulin. Why's that? Exercise pushes glucose into muscle cells by an alternative pathway that is completely independent of insulin. So the pancreas gets a bit of a break and is better primed the next time it's required to secrete insulin. In addition, exercise builds up muscle mass, providing extra space to store all the glucose that enters the blood stream after a meal. Getting thirty to sixty minutes of exercise such as walking is one of the best things you can do to lose fat, gain muscle, and bring down your blood glucose. Even a small fat loss will make a big difference to your blood glucose levels.

Ironically, untreated diabetes can cause weight loss. In fact, losing a good deal of weight rapidly is a classic symptom of type 1 diabetes. Of all the ways to lose weight, this has to be one of the worst. The absolute lack of insulin in this situation forces the body to burn fat as the only source of fuel, while levels of glucose in the blood go through the roof. A dangerous condition known as ketoacidosis can develop, because the by-products of excessive fat burning can't be excreted fast enough. Untreated, it causes coma and death.

56. Why is it that when I gain even a few pounds my blood glucose levels go up?

It's true that when you gain weight, it's harder to keep your blood glucose under control. That's because even a modest increase in body fat increases your body's resistance to the action of insulin. This hormone drives glucose out of the blood and into the cells of your body (see question 1). Your body tries hard to overcome this resistance by secreting more insulin so long as it's capable. It's a bit like shouting to make a hard-of-hearing person hear you. But many people with diabetes don't have any reserve capacity to secrete extra insulin. In other words, they can't shout any louder and they are going hoarse in the process. So blood glucose levels rise.

For this reason, there is a strong correlation between obesity and type 2 diabetes. Indeed, perhaps 80 percent or more of the people with type 2 diabetes are overweight or obese.

Type 2 diabetes results from the combination of two things: faults in insulin manufacturing and the need to secrete too much insulin, i.e., insulin resistance. Both must be present for a person to develop type 2 diabetes. To some extent both are under genetic control. Certain ethnic groups (Native Americans, Southeast Asian people) are more insulin resistant than Caucasians even when they are still young and lean. But the insulin resistance worsens as they get older—a result of lack of exercise, more body fat, and less muscle. If the insulin-secreting cells can't keep up the pace by secreting more and more insulin, then diabetes develops sooner or later.

To be honest, experts don't know if obesity causes insulin resistance, or if insulin resistance causes obesity, or if they develop independently. We do know that obesity aggravates insulin resistance. That's why gaining a pound here and there gives you higher blood glucose levels.

57. Why does my blood glucose go up when I'm sick?

Anytime that you have a cold, feel sick to your stomach, come down with the flu, go to the hospital for surgery, or are injured, you are, in a broad sense, sick. At times like these the insulin or pills that you take often become less effective for treating your diabetes.

In other words, you become more carbohydrate intolerant or insulin resistant than usual. Perhaps this is nature's way of diverting energy away from the muscles to the tissues that need it most. Experts don't really understand why. Even if you eat less food than usual, your liver keeps on releasing sugar. In fact, the longer you are without food, the more insulin resistant you become. Sometimes you will need to take extra insulin or increase the dosage of your pills. Check with your doctor.

Interestingly, recent studies have found that people undergoing any sort of surgery are better off if the required fasting period—complete abstinence from food—both before and after the surgery, is as short as possible. The longer the period without food, the slower the recovery and the greater the number of days in hospital. Of course, fasting for four to eight hours is necessary to make sure there's no food in the gut that might be vomited up during surgery. Always consult your specialist physician.

58. Can being stressed out really have something to do with my high blood sugars?

Yes, absolutely. Stress often results in elevated blood glucose levels and decreased insulin action because it is associated with the release of several counter-regulatory hormones that mobilize energy stores. This energy mobilizing effect helps people who don't have diabetes to deal better with their environment. However, people with diabetes, because of insufficient insulin availability, can't adequately metabolize stress-induced increases in blood glucose. This can lead to chronic high blood glucose levels.

Stress can also indirectly disrupt control of diabetes. When we are stressed, we often don't pay enough attention to our diet, exercise, and other ways in which we take care of ourselves.

Stress can take many forms. It can appear emotionally as anxiety, worry, or depression. Or you can experience it physically as pain and illness. Situations like a confrontation with another person or a near-miss accident can trigger the so-called fight-or-flight response and cause the release of stress hormones.

You can manage your stress. Behavioral stress management programs do work. Certain antianxiety medications also improve blood glucose control.

59. Can certain drugs increase my blood glucose levels?

There are several reports of drugs prescribed for other conditions that cause blood glucose to rise. In most cases, however, the evidence is inconclusive, because they have been reported in very few instances.

One drug that is well documented to increase blood glucose levels is a powerful steroid called prednisone, which is widely used to treat many difficult conditions. The brand names of prednisone sold in the United States are Deltasone, Liquid Pred, Meticorten, Orasone, Panasol-S, Prednicen-M, and Sterapred. If you are being treated with this powerful drug, your doctor may have to increase your doses of insulin or pills.

60. Can you tell me why my morning blood glucose reading is often higher than it was when I went to bed?

If you take insulin injections, it could be that the effect of insulin you took is waning. Your blood glucose will rise if you didn't take enough to keep your insulin level up through the night. Otherwise it is probably **the dawn phenomenon**.

The dawn phenomenon is a normal physiological process whereby certain hormones in your body work to raise blood glucose levels before you wake up. These so-called counter regulatory hormones, including glucagon, epinephrine, growth hormone, and cortisol, work against the action of insulin. They stimulate glucose release from the liver and inhibit glucose utilization throughout the body. The result is an increase in blood glucose levels, ensuring a supply of fuel in anticipation of the wakening body's needs.

It's not true that only people with type 1 diabetes experience the dawn phenomenon. People with type 2 diabetes can also experience it. Their livers continue to make new glucose even when it's not needed. In fact, even people who do not have diabetes can experience it, but for them increased insulin secretion by the pancreas keeps blood glucose levels relatively stable. The dawn phenomenon varies from person to person and can even vary from time to time in each of us.

A third—much less likely—possibility is called **the Somogyi effect** or Somogyi's phenomenon, named for an Austrian-American biochemist who first described it in 1938. The Somogyi effect can follow untreated high blood glucose in the middle of the night by causing it to go too low as a sort of rebound. You can check if this is happening by measuring if your blood glucose is low at 2 or 3 a.m. But the Somogyi effect is actually much less common than we previously thought.

What Makes My Blood Glucose Go Down?

Food Factors That Lower My Blood Glucose Levels

61. What factors in foods can make my blood glucose levels go down?

The good news is that your blood glucose will go down automatically. Assuming your body still produces insulin, your blood glucose will typically go down 40 mg/dl or so per hour following the first hour after eating a meal. A bout of exercise will make it go down faster (see question 95).

While there is nothing that you can eat or drink that will actually make your blood glucose go down in the short-term, there are a lot of foods that won't raise it much, if at all. In fact, of all the things we eat there is only one culprit that will raise your blood glucose in the short-term.

Only certain fast-acting carbohydrates—those foods with high GI values—will seriously raise your blood glucose in the short-term. Slowly digested and absorbed carbohydrates, protein, fat, fiber, and water are a much better option and won't have any impact on your blood glucose level.

It's even better news that time is on your side. If you avoid much in the way of high-glycemic carbohydrates, in the long-term your blood glucose level will be lower.

62. What effect does fat have on my blood glucose levels?

Fat consumed alone—for example, a bowl of cream—has an insignificant short-term effect on blood glucose. But combined with carbohydrate, it will slow down stomach emptying and reduce the early glycemic response to the meal. So, instant mashed potatoes have a high glycemic response, similar to pure glucose, but adding a tablespoon of butter will reduce the glucose response. That's not to say we recommend this!

While fat may not have a deleterious effect on your blood glucose levels in the short-term (a few hours), it's the long-term effect that may spell trouble. That's because fat increases insulin resistance (see question 64). When your body is insulin resistant, it has to work harder to clear carbs from the bloodstream by secreting more insulin. But some types of fat appear to be worse than others in this respect.

We should minimize the amount of saturated fat that we eat, not only to protect against heart disease, but also to optimize insulin sensitivity. Saturated fats come in all forms of fast foods, such as chicken, hamburgers, and french fries. Other sources are dairy products, fatty meats such as salamis and bacon, and cookies and cakes. You can and should eat unsaturated fats in moderate quantities. This includes the mono-unsaturated fats, such as those in olive oil and avocados, and the long-chain polyunsaturated fatty acids found in fish and shellfish. Just make sure you have them broiled, not fried!

We have learned even more recently that trans fatty acids, or trans fats, are even worse for us than saturated fats. We get most of these fats in the form of partially hydrogenated vegetable oil, which is present in 40 percent of all supermarket food products. It's in most cookies, breakfast foods, salty snacks and chips, cake mixes, and almost half of all breakfast cereals. The products with the most trans fat include vegetable shortening, doughnuts, stick margarine, french fries, and microwaved popcorn. See the box on page 96 for a breakdown of trans fatty foods.

63. What do protein foods do to my blood glucose levels?

Meat, poultry, and fish don't have any carbohydrates worth mentioning. The macronutrients in beef, lamb, pork, chicken, turkey, and fish are protein and fat.

When we eat protein foods, amino acids—the building blocks that make up protein—rise in the blood stream. About half of them are used immediately for maintenance and repair in the body. The rest are usually surplus to our needs and are simply broken down as a source of energy.

Recent studies indicate that lean protein has only a minuscule effect on elevations in blood glucose. This seems to be true for people both with and without diabetes. A 50-gram dose of protein in the form a steak (200 grams of lean beef) resulted in 10 mg/dl rise and fall in blood glucose levels.

However, if you eat some carbohydrate with your protein the story is different. We explain this synergism in the next question.

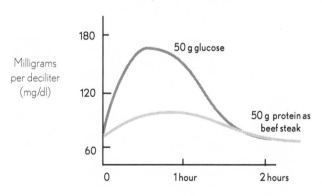

Figure 7. Blood glucose levels after a protein meal such as a piece of beef steak.

64. What happens if I eat some extra protein or fat with my carbohydrate?

Extra protein and fat will lower your overall glycemic response to a meal. There are several reasons for this. Both slow down stomach emptying and, therefore, the rate at which the carbohydrate in the meal can be digested and absorbed. Accordingly, the glycemic response will tend to be lower, but not necessarily the insulin response. In fact, chances are that the insulin response will be higher than that seen with the carbohydrate alone. This is because protein by itself stimulates insulin secretion—gram-for-gram it has about a third of the effect of pure glucose. Taken together, protein, fat, and carbohydrate tend to have a synergistic effect on insulin secretion.

The upshot of this is that a food containing a mixture of carbohydrate, fat, and protein will have a lower glycemic response than the carbohydrate alone, but the insulin response is significantly higher, and this is partly responsible for pushing glucose levels down.

Figure 8. Effect of 50 g of carbohydrate as bread with and without 50 g protein.

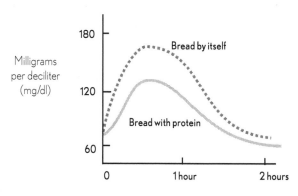

The glycemic index of the carbohydrate is still relevant in this context. If you eat some extra protein or fat with your carbohydrate, you'll still see the same relative differences among foods. For example, potatoes by themselves have a high GI value, about double that of pasta. Your potatoes with some cheese and butter will have roughly twice the glycemic effect of the same amount of carbohydrate as the pasta with cheese and butter. In other words, you can still rank your carbohydrate foods as low, moderate, and high GI when they are eaten in "mixed meals."

"The pizza effect:" If you have type 1 diabetes, you may have noticed that foods that are high in carbs as well as fat raise your blood glucose levels and then keep them there for a longer time. This might happen with a large serving of pizza or a burrito with a side of tortilla chips. In this instance, the carbs and fats are competing strongly for burning in the "engine room" of the cell, and fat's winning the race. Glucose levels are high as a result. Increasing the dose of insulin may be the best bet next time, but make sure you work off those extra calories as soon as possible.

65. What about milk and other dairy products (like cheese and yogurt), all of which have some carbohydrates?

Milk and dairy products on the whole have low blood glucose-raising abilities, even when they contain added sugar. Full-fat cow's milk has a GI value of less than 40. The average GI value of ice cream is about 60, with premium varieties being about 40. Sweetened fruit yogurts have low glycemic potencies, and artificially sweetened versions are even lower.

Dairy products are valuable additions to a low-GI diet, if you are able to tolerate lactose. Some products, such as hard yellow cheese, contain little or no lactose. Most of their energy comes from protein and fat, which means they can be consumed with impunity by lactose-intolerant individuals. For the same reason, they cannot have a GI value (only foods containing significant amounts of carbohydrate can be tested for their GI value). Essentially, you can think of cheese as having a glycemic index value of 0. The same goes for eggs, meat, and seafood.

Some soft and white cheeses contain trivial amounts of lactose, not usually enough to cause symptoms. Full-fat dairy products contain large amounts of saturated fat. For this reason, they are best kept as "indulgences," while everyday diets can contain the low fat versions.

Some investigators have found that dairy products stimulate much more insulin than their GI values would indicate. Normally, blood glucose and insulin responses are strongly correlated, but with milk and dairy products there is two to three times more insulin produced than expected for the level of glycemia. This may be because milk contains proteins and peptides or other factors that are "insulino-genic" (stimulating insulin production).

Milk is the food of all young growing mammals, and insulin is the hormone that drives uptake of all nutrients—carbohydrates, fats, and amino acids—into cells. Thus it makes sense that milk should be the perfect food for optimum deposition of new tissue and growth. However, cow's milk was designed for calves that double their birth weight within a month, compared to human infants who take several months to reach twice their birth weight. Some studies show that human milk is not as insulinogenic as cow's milk.

DAIRY PRODUCTS FROM A
BLOOD GLUCOSE PERSPECTIVE

Dairy products	Glycemic index	Glycemic load
Low-fat yogurt	14	2
Sweetened fruit yogurt	31	10
Whole milk	27	3
Skim milk	32	4
Premium ice cream	38	3
Low-fat ice cream	47	5
Condensed sweetened milk	61	17

66. But what about the long-term effect of protein and fat?

The protein and fat that you eat today won't make your blood glucose level go up today or tomorrow. However, what about the long-term? Most folks aren't concerned with it. As the economist John Maynard Keynes once quipped, "In the long run we are all dead."

Of course he's right. But if you eat enough saturated and trans fat, you might not have to wait all that long. And if your blood glucose levels are high as well, then the time bomb is ticking.

Experts are still debating the ideal proportions of fat, protein, and carbohydrate in the diet. Nevertheless, no one debates the fact that fat is more calorie-rich than anything else. Each gram of fat packs nine calories, while each gram of carbohydrate or protein has four. If you eat enough fat in any form, you can easily gain weight. But some forms of fat are good for you (see question 62) and you shouldn't throw the baby out with the bathwater. Make sure you get moderate amounts of the healthy fats found in lean meat, seafood, avocado, and olive and canola oils. Eating your salads with a small amount of olive oil and vinegar is not a crime. It not only helps to give you important fats, it helps lower blood glucose responses to the whole meal.

High-fat and high-protein diets have the potential to induce carbohydrate "intolerance." This means any carbohydrate eaten would raise blood glucose and insulin levels to greater heights on a day-to-day basis. However, even here the type of fat may be important (see question 62). A recent study shows that diets moderately high in mono-unsaturated fats (olive oil, nuts, lean meat, avocados) improved glucose tolerance, as long as the proportion of total energy as fat was not excessive, specifically not greater than 37 percent of total energy (average intakes today are less than 35 percent).

67. If protein and fat don't raise blood glucose levels, shouldn't I base my diet on them?

While it's true that protein and fat don't raise blood glucose levels, it *doesn't* necessarily follow that a high-protein–high-fat diet (in other words, a low carbohydrate diet) is best for your health. That's because human bodies are most sensitive to the hormone, insulin, when the diet contains a moderate to high amount of carbohydrate. Being insulin sensitive allows the body to metabolize the glucose in the blood with the least amount of insulin. Even lean young people will become relatively insulin resistant, if they eat a high fat or high protein diet. Insulin resistance increases the risk of obesity, cardiovascular disease, and type 2 diabetes.

Early in the last century, people with diabetes were advised to avoid carbohydrate and eat diets high in fat and protein instead. Unfortunately, they often died of heart attacks. In the late 1970s, some doctors questioned the prevailing dietary recommendations and cautiously added increasing amounts of carbohydrate to diabetic diets. To their great surprise, they found that blood glucose control improved, and **A1c** levels fell.

But these new diets were not just high in carbohydrate, they were extraordinarily high in fiber and undoubtedly *low GI.* In fact, they were so high in fiber that many Americans found them unpalatable. Thus, the main focus became a high-carbohydrate diet with only moderate amounts of fiber.

WHAT DO WE MEAN BY A1C?

Also called HbA1c, glycohemoglobin, glycated hemoglobin, or glycosylated hemoglobin, A1c is a test that measures your over-all diabetes control for the previous two to three months. The way it works is that a small amount of glucose normally binds with the hemoglobin that carries oxygen in your blood. It binds in direct proportion to the amount of glucose in your blood, and once it binds, it remains there for the lifespan of the red cell that contains hemoglobin, which is usually between two and three months.

68. What's wrong with low–carbohydrate diets?

Diets lower in carbohydrate, like those recommended by Dr. Atkins, Dr. Bernstein, and Dr. Eades, as well as *The Zone* diet, are becoming increasingly popular. Why don't we recommend them? We just don't have enough to go on yet. We need to see a lot more studies in both diabetic and non-diabetic subjects of all ethnic groups before we can recommend them.

We should be extremely cautious of diets high in saturated fats, like the Atkins diet, because of the wealth of evidence that saturated fat increases the risk of coronary heart disease in the general population. We also know that more people with diabetes died from heart disease during the period last century when low-carbohydrate diets were in vogue.

Current scientific evidence indicates that the best diet for people with diabetes is moderately high in carbohydrate (45 to 55 percent of calories). But that carbohydrate should be slowly digested and absorbed in order to help preserve insulin-secreting capacity. Type 2 diabetes develops in people who have both resistance to insulin and reduced capacity to overcome that resistance by secreting more. This means that low-GI foods are the best choice for people who have high blood glucose levels.

69. Will fish oil or flaxseed oil capsules increase my blood glucose levels or make me put on weight?

Fish oil or flaxseed oil capsules may be recommended to you for their potential to lower your cardiovascular risk. Studies have shown that the omega-3 fatty acids derived from these oils:

- Slow the buildup of fatty material on the walls of blood vessels (atherosclerosis)
- Stop the blood from becoming too thick and reduce blood clotting
- Cause a fall in triglycerides (blood fats)
- Make the arteries more elastic
- Help reduce blood pressure
- Counteract irregular heartbeat (cardiac arrhythmia).

Although some early studies suggested that fish-oil supplementation may be detrimental to blood glucose levels, the consensus from eighteen randomized, placebo-controlled trials in type 2 diabetes is that it has no significant effect on glycemic control (measured as either fasting glucose or the A1c test). Doses used in the studies ranged from 3 to 18 grams per day. Most commonly available capsules are 1,000 mg and are recommended at doses of three to six capsules per day. The 3 to 6 grams of fat this would contribute to your day (about one teaspoon or fifty calories) is unlikely to cause weight gain.

70. What effect does fiber have on my blood glucose levels? Is soluble or insoluble fiber better for me?

A high-fiber food is not necessarily one that will reduce blood glucose levels. The crucial aspect when we're talking about fiber is the form it takes in food. Insoluble fiber found in plant cell walls can have a glycemic lowering effect if it is intact in its natural form. In the coat of seeds and grains, insoluble fiber acts as a physical barrier, slowing down access of digestive enzymes to the starch inside. Pumpernickel and whole grain breads, legumes, and barley are examples where this effect is evident. All-Bran™ breakfast cereal is another example. It is made from coarsely milled wheat, which has large pieces of endosperm (starch) still attached.

Once fiber is milled, however, even if it is added back to the flour (e.g., whole wheat flour), its presence has little effect on blood glucose levels. Finely ground wheat fiber, such as that in whole wheat bread, has no effect whatsoever on the rate of starch digestion and subsequent glucose response. Products made with whole meal flour have a similar effect to that of their white flour counterparts.

Viscous or soluble fibers, on the other hand, do tend to lower blood glucose levels. They do this by increasing the viscosity of the intestinal contents, slowing the passage of food through the digestive tract, and restricting the movement of enzymes. This slows digestion and results in a lower blood glucose response. This is the case in foods like oats, legumes, and psyllium (a seed used in some breakfast cereals and laxatives).

AT-A-GLANCE:
WHAT ARE THE DIFFERENT KINDS OF FIBERS?

Fiber is an undigestable complex carbohydrate found in plants. Since the body can't absorb fiber, it has no calories. Fiber can be divided into two categories according to their physical characteristics and effects on the body: Water insoluble and water soluble. Each form functions differently and provides different health benefits.

Soluble fibers, such as gums, mucilages, and pectins, dissolve in water. They absorb water and slow the passage of food, and help to satisfy our appetite by creating a full feeling. Foods high in soluble fiber, such as oat and rice bran, oatmeal, apples, figs, barley, artichokes, and prunes, may help to reduce blood glucose. Soluble fiber may also help to reduce the level of cholesterol in the blood.

Insoluble fibers, such as cellulose, hemicellulose, and lignin, do not dissolve in water. They promote regular elimination by providing bulk for stool formation and thus hastening the passage of the stool through the colon. Foods high in insoluble fiber include dried beans, wheat bran, seeds, brown rice, and whole grain products such as breads, cereals, and pasta.

71. Can the GI values of foods predict the effect of a "mixed meal" containing lots of different foods?

Yes. You can put together a meal with foods of different glycemic index values and predict what the overall glycemic index value of the meal will be. To do this, the total carbohydrate content of the meal and the contribution of each food to the total carbohydrate must be known. This data can be obtained from food composition tables.

For example, say you have a breakfast of cornflakes with milk and sugar and a glass of orange juice. The predicted glycemic effect of this meal is calculated by multiplying the GI value of each food by the percentage of carbohydrate that it contributes to the meal, as follows:

Foods	CHO(g)	% total CHO	GI	Contribution to meal GI
Cornflakes, 1 oz.	24	51	92	51% × 92 = 47
Milk, 4 oz.	6	13	27	13% × 27 = 4
Sugar, 1 tsp	4	8	68	8% × 68 = 5
Orange juice, 4 oz.	13	28	50	28% × 50 = 14
Totals	47	100		Meal GI = 70

Obviously, meals like this aren't only a mix of carbohydrates, but include differing proportions of protein and fat as well. Nevertheless, the glycemic index value of the meal is still predictable because the quality of carbohydrate remains the same.

Why do people say that the glycemic index doesn't work with mixed meals? While over a dozen studies have shown that the glycemic index is predictable in a mixed meal context, three studies reported that it wasn't. These studies were all American (two were from the same research group), and their negative findings were well publicized, but the researchers did not follow the standard GI testing procedure.

A FEW WORDS ABOUT MIXED MEALS

In the United States, the original criticism of the glycemic index was based on two factors, one of which was that the glycemic index did not work in a mixed meal context. However, this objection no longer prevails.

Three well-publicized American studies found that the glycemic index does not apply to mixed meals, but the fine detail shows that the investigators who conducted the studies did not use the standardized methodology for glycemic index testing. Instead of using the fasting blood glucose level to determine the area under the curve, they used a baseline of 0 mg/dl. This makes no sense to us because 1) a blood glucose reading of 0 is impossibly low, and 2) we are interested in the *fluctuation* of blood glucose levels, not the area below "sea level." Over a dozen other studies have proven that the GI values can, in fact, be measured for mixed meals.

Even the American Diabetes Association (ADA) says that low-GI foods help reduce blood sugar levels after we eat. A recent meta-analysis—in which multiple studies involving the glycemic index were analyzed—has shown there are small but clinically useful improvements in glycemic control in people with type 1 and type 2 diabetes.

72. How much water should I drink?

The big advantage of water over just about anything else that we drink is that it has a glycemic index of zero. It won't raise your blood sugar at all.

But it's not true that you have to drown yourself in the stuff. There's an old urban myth that you should drink at least eight glasses of water a day. While you will see this advice repeated time and again, it appears to lack any scientific proof.

It looks like the Food and Nutrition Board of the National Research Council started the whole thing in 1945. That's when the board recommended that we consume about "1 milliliter of water for each calorie of food." That works out to roughly 2–2½ quarts per day. But most people seem to have missed its next sentence, that "most of this quantity is contained in prepared foods."

Fruits and vegetables in particular give us a lot of the water we need. They are 80 to 95 percent water. This is in addition to the juices, milk, and other beverages we consume.

Where does that leave us? When you are thirsty, water remains your best choice. Even when you are hungry, having a drink of water is a great idea. It can help you feel fuller and therefore make you less likely to overeat. This will go a long way toward keeping your blood sugar under control.

73. Does coffee or tea affect my blood glucose?

Coffee in particular remains one of the favorite whipping boys of the food police. In study after study, coffee and its caffeine content are blamed for everything from high blood pressure, high cholesterol, and increased homocysteine levels to ulcers and painful burns.

Some of these effects may indeed be real. However, one certainly isn't. Neither coffee nor tea will raise your blood glucose.

One American diabetes magazine in a review of the first (Australian) edition of *The New Glucose Revolution* wrote that "morning coffee" had a glycemic index value of 79. They overlooked the heading that explained that it was a brand of cookies sold in Australia.

You do drink coffee or tea straight, don't you? If, however, you drink it with milk or cream or sugar, those additives will have their normal effect in raising your blood glucose.

74. What effect will diet beverages have on my blood glucose?

Diet beverages basically consist of water, colors, flavors, and noncaloric sweeteners. Some diet fruit beverages with 5 percent fruit juice will contain trace amounts of carbohydrate, but such small amounts will not affect your blood glucose levels. Diet beverages are also very low calorie and are therefore considered a "free food" for those with diabetes.

This is not a license to go overboard. While diet beverages don't contain fermentable carbohydrates, they are still associated with erosion of tooth enamel. This is because their high acidity dissolves calcium and, when sipped frequently, can increase the risk of tooth decay.

75. Is it safe for me to use noncaloric sweeteners such as sucralose, stevia, and aspartame?

Noncaloric sweeteners are just that—noncaloric—meaning they provide no energy. They are hundreds of times sweeter than sugar, but will not affect your blood glucose levels or your weight. Aspartame (i.e., NutraSweet™) is slightly different in that it contains four calories per gram, but is used in such minute quantities that it can be considered noncaloric. Sucralose itself has no calories. But the granular Splenda™ has four calories per gram that come from maltodextrin, which is added to provide bulk.

Noncaloric sweeteners are classed as food additives, and approval for their inclusion in foods is regulated by the U.S. Food and Drug Administration (FDA). The FDA considers stevia an unapproved food additive, so it cannot be promoted as a sweetener, but under provisions of 1994 legislation it can be sold as a "dietary supplement."

A safe level of intake is expressed as an acceptable daily intake (ADI), which is an amount per kilogram of body weight that a person can safely consume every day over a lifetime without risk. The ADI is usually an amount one hundred times less than the maximum level at which no observed adverse effect occurs in animal studies. The general population consumes noncaloric sweeteners at levels below 10 percent of the ADI. While people with diabetes may be higher consumers, their levels of intake could be considered safe.

76. What does alcohol do to my blood glucose levels? Does different alcohol—beer, wine, liquor—have different effects?

In our studies, we've found that an alcoholic beverage, consumed alone, reduced both glucose and insulin levels in lean, young, and healthy subjects. This was the case with beer, wine, or liquor. Beer contains some carbohydrate, but the amount present is small, and the initial rise in blood glucose levels is followed by a return to baseline levels and below. When the drinks were served with a carbohydrate meal, glucose and insulin responses were again lower compared with the meal given with water. These findings are not surprising, because it is well known that alcohol inhibits the production of new glucose molecules in the liver. In fact, after a heavy night of drinking, people can wake up with such low glucose levels that their exercise performance is compromised. In people with diabetes taking insulin, severe life-threatening hypoglycemia can develop if they consume a few drinks without an accompanying meal or snack.

Figure 9. Comparison of bread, beer, wine or spirits (240 calories of each) on blood glucose levels.

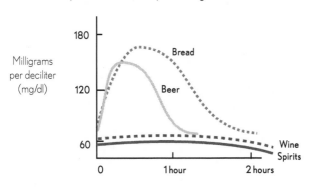

Alcoholic beverages have also been associated with reduced risk of cardiovascular disease. Those who drink one to three standard drinks a day have lower risk than teetotalers. However, with consumption of five or more drinks, risk again increases. Scientists have found that alcohol increases levels of the good cholesterol, HDL. But some of this favorable effect could be due to lowering of blood glucose and insulin levels.

Our take home message: *Drink in moderation, if at all*— zero to three drinks per day, with one or two alcohol-free days per week.

77. Since food makes my blood glucose levels go up, wouldn't fasting be the best way to bring it down?

We know that too much exposure to the sun can cause skin cancer. In which case, you might conclude that the best way to avoid skin cancer would be to live in a cave. The trouble is, you would develop rickets from lack of sun. When you go to extremes, you can run into other problems.

Fasting certainly will bring down blood glucose levels. Particularly if you get insulin shots or take certain medications for type 2 diabetes, fasting, in fact, can take your blood glucose levels too low. The resulting hypoglycemia can be both uncomfortable and dangerous.

Fasting increases insulin resistance and forces your liver to manufacture all the glucose needed by the brain all by itself. If you have type 2 diabetes, that ability can be impaired. In particular, fasting requires your liver to release glucose into the blood in order to keep your brain and other organs going. Once all the stored glucose has gone—which normally takes only a matter of hours—the liver will start making new glucose molecules. Your body will start breaking down muscle proteins to provide the carbon atoms needed. In itself, that's not a problem, but if you have type 2 diabetes, the liver often doesn't know when to stop and releases way too much glucose. Consequently, your blood glucose levels may run high for quite some time.

This doesn't mean that fasting is completely out of the question. Many people with diabetes fast to participate in religious events. While they usually have the option of avoiding a fast if necessary to preserve their health, they are often happier if they are able to participate without adversely affecting control of their diabetes. Usually, your doctor and you will be able to work out a plan tailor-made for your circumstances.

78. Which carbohydrates will raise my blood glucose the least?

This is another way of asking the question, which foods have low GI values? We can summarize them here, but there are too many to list all of them. You can look up the GI value of a food in the tables at the back of this book.

Ironically, many vegetables that have little protein or fat also have too little carbohydrate to test for their GI values. These are the so-called "free foods," which we address fully in question 84. This includes most of what we think of as the green vegetables, but also includes everything from cabbage and cauliflower to tomatoes and turnips.

Of all the foods tested for their GI values, no group scores lower than legumes—which includes beans, lentils, and peas. Lowest of all legumes is chana dal, which is especially popular in India. You can read about it and find many recipes at www.mendosa.com/chanadal.html.

The world's most important vegetables are rice, corn, and wheat. These are the staple crops for most people.

Different types of rice have perhaps the greatest glycemic variability of any food. The type with the least blood glucose impact is one commonly available in U.S. supermarkets—Uncle Ben's parboiled (converted) rice.

Corn, corn on the cob, and corn tortillas contain low-GI carbs. Strangely, popcorn contains quickly digested carbs, probably because the puffing makes all the starch easier to break down.

Wheat kernels and pasta contain low-GI starches. Semolina or cracked wheat is the starting point for making most traditional pastas. But most everything made from wheat flour, including wheat bread, crackers, cookies, and breakfast cereals, have high GI values. The difference is the particle size—smaller particles mean a higher glycemic response.

Of all the grains, barley will have the least effect on your blood glucose. Pearled barley, the form in which we usually eat it, lacks the bran. Nevertheless, no other cereal crop has ever been tested with a lower GI. Hull-less barley, in which the bran is left intact, probably has an even lower glycemic index, but it hasn't been tested.

Oatmeal, known elsewhere as porridge, has a moderate effect on blood glucose, as does oat bran.

79. Should we avoid foods, like soybeans, that are high in anti-nutrients even if they have positive effects on blood glucose?

Definitely not. **Anti-nutrients** are a wide variety of substances present naturally in foods that are able to bind enzymes or nutrients and thereby block the action or absorption of nutrients. Anti-nutrients are part of the plant's arsenal of chemicals designed to deter insects and other predators. Common ones are protease inhibitors, amylase inhibitors, phytic acid, and polyphenolic compounds such as tannins. With proper soaking and germination or cooking, none of these are anything to worry about.

Some anti-nutrients, like the phytoestrogens, are now considered in a completely new light. Soybeans are the richest source of flavonoids. Many experts attribute the low risk of breast cancer in Asian countries specifically to the consumption of soybeans.

Iron deficiency anemia correlates best with low intakes of heme iron, not with phytic acid intake.

Until a hundred years ago, the Pima Indians of Arizona were the world's largest consumers of legumes, one of the highest sources of anti-nutrients. The Pimas recognized the importance of long cooking times and, interestingly, diabetes was absent. Now they eat mostly American food and have the highest rates of diabetes in the world.

80. I thought that carrots had a big effect on blood glucose. Why are they now considered okay?

Ever since the first foods were tested for their blood glucose-raising capability, we have had questions about whether to eat carrots or not. The first journal article ever published on this indicated that we quickly digest the carbohydrates in carrots. We now suspect that value was wrong.

The original study tested only five instead of the usual 10 or more subjects. There was also two to three times more variation among the subjects who tested carrots than other foods in that study.

More recent careful studies at the University of Sydney and elsewhere now show that carrots and carrot juice have quite low GI values. Cooked carrots have a mean GI value of 47 in four studies. The one study of raw carrot juice returned a GI value of 43.

Some might see this "back-flip" on carrots as evidence of the unreliability of the GI concept. But GI testing is now a standardized procedure and we know a lot more about why results have varied. It's important to have at least eight subjects and to have tested the reference food in each subject two to three times, so that we have a good picture of day-to-day variation in glucose tolerance. These standards were not applied in the first test of carrots. Just like we wouldn't expect every hamburger to be 35 percent fat, we shouldn't expect the glycemic index to be precisely the same in each individual. But the average fat content of a hamburger is still a valuable figure to know. And the same applies to the glycemic index—you can expect that the average value will apply to you, *on average*.

81. Will a big salad have a marked effect on my blood glucose levels?

Too often, salad is treated as the garnish that's left behind on the plate after the main dish has been eaten. But that pile of greens deserves more consideration. First, there is the big advantage that none of the usual ingredients in vegetable salad will have much of an effect on your blood glucose. Given its negligible calorie content as well, salad automatically qualifies as something to be eaten liberally by people with diabetes.

Adding a little pasta to your salad won't make your blood glucose level rise sharply. High-protein ingredients like hard cheese, cottage cheese, or canned tuna will also have little or no effect.

WHAT ABOUT CHICKPEA SALAD AND BEAN SALAD?

The salads that have the least effects on your blood glucose levels are the big leafy vegetable type, but chickpea and bean salads deserve a special mention. Both of these salads are rich in low GI carbohydrate and protein, so they stand alone as excellent, satisfying meals with favorable effects on blood glucose levels.

If you do eat salad liberally, you'll experience another advantage—it feels filling. Your stomach is satisfied with its capacity being occupied by fiber and water. Next comes the nutrients—you get loads more water-soluble vitamins like folate and vitamin C than in cooked vegetables, plus the hidden benefits of phytonutrients like lycopene, which is in tomatoes. And finally, salad with a meal provides a medium for you to use some vinaigrette, which, as we explain in the next question, can lower the glycemic impact of your entire meal.

While croutons make a crunchy garnish for salads, they do contain carbohydrate, which may affect blood glucose. A small handful could easily supply 10 grams of carbohydrate, which is likely to raise your blood glucose level. So don't be too heavy-handed with them.

Potato salad is something else entirely. Because potatoes have such a great capacity to raise your blood glucose level, it's better to skip the potato salad.

82. What are the advantages of eating vinegar, lemon juice, and sourdough bread?

Physiologists have long known that highly acidic solutions slow down stomach emptying. The surprise, however, is how little is needed to reduce blood glucose levels. Several studies have shown that a realistic amount of vinegar or lemon juice, in the form of a salad dressing, consumed with a mixed meal has significant blood glucose lowering effects. For example, 4 teaspoons of vinegar in a vinaigrette dressing (4 teaspoons vinegar and 8 teaspoons oil) taken with an average meal lowered blood glucose by as much as 30 percent. These findings have important implications for people with diabetes or individuals at risk of diabetes, coronary heart disease, or Syndrome X (also known as the metabolic syndrome) (impaired glucose tolerance, hypertension, and high blood lipid levels).

The effect appears to be related to the acidity, because other organic acids (such as lactic acid and propionic acid) also have a blood glucose lowering effect. However, the degree of reduction varies with the type of acid. Acids that are small molecules work best. Thus hydrochloric acid—the acid secreted by the cells in your stomach to kick-start the digestion process—is the best. But don't even consider taking hydrochloric acid by mouth—it will burn the lining of the mouth, throat, and esophagus beyond repair.

Our studies have shown that lemon juice is just as powerful as vinegar. Lime juice is likely to work just as well. Acidic fruits such as passion fruit will also do the trick, but the more sugar they contain, the less likely an effect will be seen, because the two things will cancel each other out.

Our take-home message: A side salad with your meal is a good habit to get into (the French and Italians do it all the time).

Sourdough breads, in which lactic acid and propionic acid are produced by the natural fermentation of starch and sugars by the yeast starter culture, also produce levels of blood glucose and insulin 22 percent lower than non-sourdough bread. In addition, there was higher satiety associated with breads having decreased rates of digestion and absorption. Thus, there is significant potential to lower blood glucose and insulin and increase satiety with sourdough bread formulations.

83. I heard that cooked cactus pads are a good diabetic food item. Is that right?

Prickly pear cactus (*Opuntia* sp.), also known as nopal or nopalitos, is, in Mexican folklore, reputed to reduce blood glucose. The pads of this cactus are the part most commonly eaten, although they have forbidding spines that have to be removed first. Available bagged and cleaned in Mexican markets and bottled in many supermarkets, particularly in the Southwest, prickly pear cactus is often eaten in salads, as a side vegetable, or with eggs.

It contains pectin and other fiber components that may have hypoglycemic activity. A few studies reported in peer-reviewed journals have shown this cactus to reduce blood glucose. However, most have been small, uncontrolled trials published only in Spanish or dealing with animals (the non-human variety).

Whether or not prickly pear cactus will make your blood glucose go down in the long-term, it is clear that it won't make it go up after a meal. It has been tested for its GI value, which is very low—only 7.

84. Why are there so few vegetables on the lists of GI values?

Many vegetables have few available carbohydrates in a standard serving. We call these the "free foods," not because your supermarket will give them to you without cost, but because they are essentially free of any impact on your blood glucose.

Another factor is that, because servings of these vegetables are so low in available carbohydrates, it's difficult, if not impossible, to get volunteers to eat enough for a test. The standard test portion is 50 grams of available carbohydrates. With any of the free foods, test subjects would have to eat huge portions.

For convenience, we can call any vegetable with fewer than 5 grams of available carbohydrate in a 100 gram portion a free food. The rest of the portion is protein, fat, fiber, ash, and water.

You can find many of these vegetables in the USDA Nutrient Database for Standard Reference on the Internet. The most common ones are:

- Asparagus
- Broccoli
- Cabbage and sauerkraut
- Celeriac
- Celery
- Cucumber
- Eggplant
- Fennel
- Green beans

- Greens (including collards, kale, mustard, parsley, purslane, spinach, swiss chard, and tops from beets and turnips)
- Jicama
- Lettuce (all types including arugula, endive, radicchio, and watercress)
- Mushrooms (all types except shitake)
- Nopales
- Okra
- Peppers (both sweet and hot)
- Radishes
- Scallions (green onions)
- Sprouted alfalfa seeds
- Summer squash (including zucchini)
- Tomatillos
- Tomatoes and tomato juice
- Turnips

In addition, three fruits—avocados, raspberries, and strawberries—have fewer than 5 grams of available carbohydrate per 100 gram portion. Likewise, two nuts—macadamias and pecans—can also be counted among the free foods. Just remember that the avocados and the nuts are high in fat.

85. What about spices—can they affect blood glucose levels? I've heard that cinnamon helps lower blood glucose while black pepper raises it. Is that correct?

It's conceivable that some spices contain bioactive substances that alter glucose metabolism, just like diabetes medications.

Researchers at the U.S. Department of Agriculture's Human Nutrition Research Center in Beltsville, Maryland, have tested about fifty plant extracts for their effects on glucose metabolism. One of them—cinnamon—increased glucose uptake about twenty times in test tube assays of fat cells. None of the other plants tested so far come close.

Led by Agricultural Research Service chemist, Dr. Richard A. Anderson, the researchers subsequently confirmed their findings with human subjects.

They tried all the different species of cinnamon, and they all had a similar effect, he says. So too did numerous commercial bottles of cinnamon.

There is one red flag: The Dutch health and food newsletter *Gezond* recently published an article about the risks of coumarin, one of the flavorings in cinnamon. In animal studies, coumarin causes mutations or cancer.

However, essentially all toxic materials in cinnamon are insoluble, Dr. Anderson says. Therefore, he uses a water-soluble extract.

He recommends taking ¼ to 1 teaspoon daily. If you want to take more, boil the cinnamon in water and pour off the soluble portion and discard the solid cinnamon.

Increasing the amount of cinnamon that you eat won't cure your diabetes. But it could reduce how much insulin or oral medications you need. That means you will need to test even more often.

In Japan the so-called Low Insulin Diet has become quite a craze. You can read about it in many books. One of these books shows a very high glycemic index for black pepper. That's no doubt incorrect.

The first problem is that there is no possible way that black pepper could have been tested with the standard method. As we've previously discussed, normally ten or more volunteers eat 50 grams of available carbohydrate of the test food and compare the results against what happens when they take the same amount of glucose. In some cases, 25 grams of available carbohydrate are used. However, testing even 5 grams (a whole teaspoon) of black pepper is unthinkable.

Bear in mind that even the precise legal profession uses cutoff values below which lawyers don't concern themselves. They call this *de minimis.* It's a short way of expressing the Latin phrase, *de minimis non curat lex* (the law does not concern itself with trifles). The amount of black pepper that anyone uses is so small as to have essentially no effect on anyone's blood glucose levels.

86. Is it true that pineapple juice has less effect on blood glucose levels than pineapple?

It sounds unlikely, doesn't it? After all, juices have a smaller particle size than whole fruits. And generally, a smaller particle size means a higher glycemic value. But a direct comparison between the GI values listed for juice versus fresh pineapple is not scientifically valid, given the different origins of the pineapples—in this case the products were from different countries. Unless the same batch of fruit is used to make the juice, it's quite possible that differences in acidity and type of sugar (ripeness) will affect the final glycemic response.

We have tests for three other fruits and juices made from them—apples and apple juice, grapefruit and grapefruit juice, and oranges and orange juice. In each of these cases the juice is more glycemic than the whole fruit. Still, all rank as low glycemic foods.

We recommend that you try to eat whole fruits whenever possible, because they are more satiating than the juice and much less likely to be overeaten. If you enjoy a glass of juice, keep it small—about 4 ounces.

87. I've heard that it's better for me to eat dried apricots than fresh apricots. Is that true? It doesn't make sense to me, because dried apricots are more concentrated.

Some people have assumed that dried apricots are better than fresh ones because the dried fruit has a lower GI value. It's true that *one* dried apricot will have less effect than *one* fresh apricot, but let's consider average serving sizes. The rise in our blood glucose depends on both the GI value of the food and the amount of carbohydrate in the serving, i.e., the glycemic load (see question 29). A normal serving of fresh apricots would be three to four apricots, containing about 9 grams of carbohydrate, giving a glycemic load value of 5. Compare this to a serving of dried apricots, say a handful, or 2 ounces. This amount of dried apricots yields about 30 grams of carbohydrate, so the GL value is 9— almost double that of the fresh product. This means that a normal serving of dried apricots will, in fact, raise your blood glucose levels more than a normal serving of fresh ones.

This still leaves the question, why do dried apricots have a lower GI value than fresh ones? Apricots are high in fructose (about half their carbohydrate), which has a low GI. The chewy, compact structure of dried apricots probably limits the access of digestive enzymes and could account for their lower GI. This appears to be the case with prunes (dried plums) and dried apples, as well.

88. How can some fruit, like dates, raise my blood glucose dramatically, while others, like cherries, have hardly any effect?

The difference between dates and cherries is certainly wide, but it is probably not as wide as you think. The reported GI value of 103 for dates is based on preliminary unpublished observations from just one study. More recent research indicates that their GI value may be much lower (less than 50), at least for some varieties of dates.

Likewise, the reported GI value of 22 for cherries is based on just one study on sour German cherries. That study is suspect because it dates from the 1970s, before we standardized glycemic index testing, and because some other foods they tested then differ considerably from tests of those foods done later. In fact, a recent Australian study suggests that those red ripe cherries we are most familiar with have a GI value of around 60.

There are still wide differences between some fruits—watermelon, for example has a glycemic index of over 70, while apples are around 40. We think the difference arises because of the water content of the fruit—the more dilute the sugars in the fruit, as in watermelon, the faster they empty from the stomach and the faster they are absorbed. This effect might also explain why fresh fruit can have a higher glycemic index than the dried version.

89. Some people tell me that watermelon sends blood glucose levels soaring, but others say that's wrong. What's the truth?

The truth is that a normal serving of watermelon won't have much effect on blood glucose levels. Those who've got it wrong are taking the high GI value of watermelon in isolation. It's important to consider the amount of carbohydrate in a normal serving as well as the GI value. Watermelon and other melons such as cantaloupe are high GI value foods, but are relatively "dilute" sources of carbohydrate. They have only about 5 percent available carbohydrate, which makes their glycemic load low. A low glycemic load means minimal impact on your blood glucose levels. Both melons, in moderate servings, are an excellent snack.

Some people think these examples make the GI concept less useful. However, in reality, there are *very few* common foods with a high GI value/low GL. Broad beans, pumpkin, and turnips are in this category too. Generally, you can rely on the glycemic index of a food to be a good guide to its effect on blood glucose levels—as long as it's consumed in typical quantities.

90. What can I snack on? What snacks won't adversely affect my blood glucose level?

For all around health benefits, fruit would have to be one of the healthiest snacks around. Although GI values for fruit range from 22 (for cherries) to 103 (for dates), the glycemic load of a standard serving of fresh fruit varies from 1 (for strawberries) to 12 (for bananas). Many fruits, such as apples, apricots, kiwi fruit, oranges, peaches, pears, plums, and melons, have GL values from 4 to 6.

Dried fruit is also a healthy, sweet snack, but is more concentrated in carbohydrate, so the GL value can be high unless the serving size is kept small. Prunes, for example, have a nice low GI of 29, and around ten prunes (2 ounces.) have a GL of 10.

For a low carbohydrate snack which won't put your blood glucose up, you shouldn't overlook nuts. Although high in fat and, therefore, in total calories, regular nut consumption is associated with better cardiovascular health. This is attributable to a number of characteristics, including the predominance of poly and monounsaturated fats, antioxidants, and dietary fiber.

Of course, free foods like salad vegetables—tomatoes, carrots, radishes, cucumbers, red peppers, green beans, and freshly shelled peas—are excellent low calorie snacks that are full of nutrition and have little impact on blood glucose levels.

91. What are the "sinful snacks" that won't raise my blood glucose too much?

"Everything in moderation" and "A little of what you like won't hurt" are good rules of thumb to keep in mind when answering this question. You can use your knowledge of the glycemic index of foods and the glycemic load of your serving to help in choosing something that won't raise your blood glucose too much. To put your knowledge into practice, remember these points:

If your snack's serving doesn't contain much carbohydrate, then it doesn't really matter if it is high or low-glycemic. It is likely to have a low glycemic load, and therefore less of an impact on your blood glucose level. For example, cantaloupe is only 5 percent carbohydrate. A slice of cantaloupe has an intermediate GI value (65) but contains very little carbohydrate (only 6 grams per 120-gram serving) so its GL value is a low 4.

On the other hand, sugar is 100 percent carbohydrate, but your serving size may be small. A teaspoon of sugar has an intermediate GI value (68), but provides only about 4 grams of carbohydrate, making its GL value 3.

If your serving is fairly substantial in terms of the amount of carbohydrate, the GI value is quite significant. For example, two donuts have a high GI value (76), and a standard serving provides about 50 grams of carbohydrate, making the GL value a whopping 38.

Low glycemic snack choices are:

▶ A peanut butter and chocolate chip snack bar—This has a low GI (37) and, with about 30 grams of carbohydrate per bar, the GL value is 10.

- A serving of ice cream—This has a GI value of about 60, and a scoop in a small cone contains about 15 grams of carbohydrate, giving it a GL value of 9.
- A cup of plain yogurt—This has a GI value of 36, but a 200-gram cup contains only 9 grams of carbohydrate, making the GL value only 3. You could add a little honey (GI=55) or some of your favorite jam (GI=24 to 36) and increase the GL value by another 3 units.
- A wedge of hard cheese—It has so little carbohydrate that the glycemic index is effectively zero.
- A hard-boiled egg—Its glycemic index is effectively zero. The eggs enriched with omega-3 fats are best.

Of course, while these choices may be okay as far as your blood glucose goes, they may not be ideal in terms of fat and other dietary considerations. So moderation and occasional frequency—choosing something you really enjoy—is the key.

92. Can I eat nuts and seeds in moderation?

Yes. Nuts and seeds are nutritious foods. They are high in protein and fiber, and many are good sources of vitamin E, zinc, magnesium, calcium, and some B-group vitamins. All nuts, except chestnuts, are high in fat, but are predominantly mono and polyunsaturated. Walnuts, pecans, and flaxseeds have the bonus of containing omega-3 fats. Research suggests that consuming a small handful of nuts (about 1 ounce) on most days of the week is beneficial in lowering cholesterol and reducing the risk of heart attack. The downside concerns anyone who is watching their weight. Their high fat content makes nuts an energy-dense food, which means as little as a tiny handful (¼ cup) provides as many calories as four slices of bread.

Nuts (except chestnuts) contain little carbohydrate, so they have negligible effects on blood glucose levels. Peanuts and cashews contain slightly more carbohydrate, but the GI values of peanuts (14) and of cashews (22) are still low.

For anyone (except those with an allergy) nuts and seeds in moderation can make a nutritious and tasty contribution to your diet. You may like to:

▶ Add a handful of toasted cashews or sesame seeds to stir-fry vegetables.
▶ Spread bread with peanut butter, almond butter, tahini, or avocado, rather than butter or margarine.
▶ Sprinkle a mixture of peanuts, flaxseeds, or sunflower seeds over cereal or salads or add to baked goods like muffins.

Nuts are an excellent snack for anyone trying to gain weight and for lean, active people who want something satisfying that has little impact on their blood glucose levels. They make a far healthier snack than potato chips, chocolate, or cookies.

NUTS AND SEEDS

Caution: Nuts and seeds are not recommended in the diet of a young child because of the risk of choking. Any nut product is best not introduced until after the first 12 months of life because of the high risk of allergy.

Non-Food Factors That Lower My Blood Glucose Levels

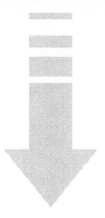

93. What can I do to bring down my blood glucose levels when they're high?

You may have been taught how to correct low blood glucose levels, but we're often asked what you can do when your levels are up.

We need to qualify our answer to this question in terms of the situation in which you find your blood glucose levels are up. First of all, if your blood glucose levels are generally under control and you get the occasional elevated reading, say from overeating, following are the things you could do:

- ▶ Do nothing. Given time, your blood glucose levels will come back down.
- ▶ Get some exercise. Physical activity consumes glucose and enhances the action of insulin, which will work to lower your blood glucose levels.
- ▶ Take extra insulin. If you take insulin to manage your diabetes, you may interpret an elevated reading as an indication of the need for some extra short-acting insulin. Bear in mind that regularly upping your insulin dose because you overate is a sure way to put on weight.
- ▶ Relax. For some people, just worrying about something can bring their blood glucose levels up. That's because the stress hormones, such as cortisol, raise blood glucose levels in preparation for fight-or-flight. If this is the case for you, address the worry or take your mind off it—say, by taking a long walk.

If, on the other hand, your blood glucose levels are consistently too high—above 140 mg/dl—then some longer-term strategies may need to be considered. The longer-term strategies that may help to lower your blood glucose levels include:

- A low glycemic index diet. Reducing the GI value of your diet can lower your blood glucose levels and increase your body's sensitivity to insulin.
- Weight loss. If you are overweight, weight loss can improve your body's sensitivity to insulin.
- Medication. Oral hypoglycemic agents or insulin may be prescribed by your doctor to lower your blood glucose levels.
- Stress management. Living a chronically stressed lifestyle may contribute to elevated blood glucose levels, so a stress management course, counseling, relaxation therapy, or a reassessment of your overall lifestyle may be in order.

94. How much exercise should a person with diabetes do?

The short answer is, as much as you can.

There is overwhelming evidence that increased levels of physical activity are of tremendous benefit to the management of diabetes—and health in general, for that matter.

Regular, moderate-intensity exercise:

▶ Helps keep blood glucose levels under control
▶ Reduces blood pressure
▶ Increases HDL or good cholesterol
▶ Helps with weight control

New recommendations from the Institute of Medicine at the National Academy of Sciences suggest adults and children aim to spend at least one hour each day in moderately intense physical activity, but this need not be all at once. A suitable level of intensity would be one that increases your rate of breathing, but still enables you to talk normally. If you need to lose weight, there is evidence that the intensity needs to be a little greater, so that even talking is difficult.

Of course, increasing the amount of exercise you do should be approached gradually. If you don't usually exercise, a medical check up is advisable before you begin.

EXERCISE

Moderate exercise is a great way to lower your blood glucose levels. Exercise is often said to have an insulin-like effect because it stimulates our muscles to take up glucose. It also makes our cells more sensitive to insulin so that the benefits continue for hours after the exercise.

95. Will exercise always lower my blood glucose level?

There are certain situations where your efforts with exercise may backfire and increase your blood glucose level instead of lowering it.

One of these is if the exercise is too strenuous and therefore stressful to your body. In this case the release of stress hormones, which antagonize the action of insulin and stimulate glucose release from body stores, will increase your blood glucose levels.

The other situation is if you have type 1 diabetes and your blood glucose level was too high before you started exercising. Your high blood glucose level reflects a relative shortage of insulin in your body, so even though your exercising muscles want to burn up glucose, there isn't sufficient insulin available to move the glucose into them. For this reason, those with type 1 diabetes are advised against exercise if their fasting blood glucose level is above 250 mg/dl and **ketosis** is present. People with type 1 diabetes should use caution—don't start exercising if your blood glucose level is above 300 mg/dl, ketosis or not.

WHAT IS KETOSIS?

You have ketosis when you have too many ketones in your body. Ketones are intermediate products in the oxidation of fat to energy, and they are synthesized in the liver. Our bodies normally use ketones at the same rate that they are produced. But, when insulin is in very short supply, the rate of production exceeds the rate of usage and the concentration in the blood rises. This results in the condition known as ketosis.

96. How do the pills that lower my blood glucose work?

In people with type 2 diabetes, when diet and exercise fail to control blood glucose levels, one or more types of drugs and/or insulin may be recommended. There are six classes of diabetes drugs that work in different ways to lower blood glucose levels.

The first class consists of what are known as **sulfony-lureas**, which work by stimulating your pancreas to make a bit more insulin. This sometimes causes them to have the side effect of causing low blood glucose, or hypoglycemia, and they can also increase body weight if used at high doses for long periods. Some examples are glimepiride (Amaryl) and glipizide (Glucotrol).

Another much newer class of drugs are the **megli-tinides**, such as repaglinide (Prandin), and a closely related class, an amino acid D-phenylalanine derivative, nateglin-ide (Starlix). These increase insulin secretion by similar means to the sulfonylureas, but they have a shorter duration of action. This means you take the pill just before you eat and it works right away, and then runs out, making it less likely to cause hypoglycemia.

Biguanides are another class of drug. The generic name for the only form of this drug available in the United States is metformin (marketed as either Glucophage or generic metformin). Biguanides are often described as making insulin work better, and one of the ways they do this is by increasing the sensitivity of the body to insulin. Because of this they may be used to complement the action of sul-fonylureas. They have other benefits as well, including pre-vention of weight gain, reducing triglycerides and possibly LDL-cholesterol, and some other vascular effects that can improve cardiovascular outcome. One disadvantage is the gastrointestinal side effects that some people experience with metformin.

Yet another class of medications works by delaying carbohydrate digestion. Acarbose (Precose) and miglitol (Glyset) are examples of alpha-glucosidase inhibitors which delay the absorption of glucose from the gastrointestinal tract. This means they can lower blood glucose levels after meals. Unfortunately, side effects like flatulence and diarrhea are common with these drugs.

Another newer class of diabetes drugs is the **thiazolidinediones**. These improve glycemic control by decreasing insulin resistance and decreasing the liver's production of glucose. Examples are rosiglitazone (marketed as Avandia) and pioglitazone (marketed as Actos). These pills can cause weight gain in the first year of use, but are usually well tolerated and don't cause hypoglycemia.

97. How can I avoid ever needing insulin?

This question stems from one of the greatest fears many people have about diabetes—injecting insulin. Of course, those with type 1 diabetes don't have any choice—insulin has to be a part of everyday life—but with type 2 diabetes insulin therapy is frequently seen as the last resort when diet, exercise, and pills have failed. But avoiding insulin at all costs is not in your best interest. In fact, if it were considered sooner rather than later, the risk of complications would be much lower and your quality of life would be higher. Very often your capacity to secrete insulin may be compromised right from the time of diagnosis. If that capacity is very low, your blood glucose levels will be high despite all your best efforts. So using an outside source of insulin lends a helping hand.

The majority of insulin used by people with diabetes is identical to and works in exactly the same way as that made by the body. These days, there is an alternative to drawing up and injecting insulin with a syringe. Insulin pens make taking insulin quicker and easier. They look something like a large ballpoint pen with a screw-on needle (in place of the point), a cartridge of insulin (much like the ink refill), and a mechanism for dialing up the dose. What's more, insulin injections are now next to painless, with much less "ouch" than your normal fingerprick blood glucose testing. So be brave and give it a go.

Insulin pumps, another way to deliver insulin to your body, are increasingly popular for people with type 1 diabetes. They deliver a basal level of insulin at a steady rate throughout the day. For mealtimes, precise amounts can be administered to match the carbohydrate in the meal. Lastly, inhaled insulin—delivered by a device similar to that used by asthmatics—is under clinical trial at present. It won't be long before insulin is "ouchless."

98. Are there any forms of alternative medicine that can lower my blood glucose?

Some people report lower blood glucose after taking certain minerals and other alternative treatments such as traditional Chinese medicine, Ayurvedic remedies, and holistic medications. None of these have been subjected to rigorous testing or have a standardized dose. And because you can't know how much of any active ingredients you are getting, it is difficult to know how much to take, particularly if you are also using insulin or oral drugs to reduce your blood glucose. In addition, there may be other components present that are not desirable, such as the toxic metals, mercury and cadmium. There are no laws covering the purity or composition of alternative medicines, and practioners can do what they like.

Alternative diabetes treatments need to be supported by good scientific studies.

Scientific support is the hallmark of Western medicine. The standards of these studies keep rising, and to be well accepted, a study must be randomized, placebo controlled, and double blind. In other words, volunteers must be assigned in a random fashion to either the dummy pill (placebo) or the test substance, and neither they nor their clinician should be aware of which is which (they are both "blinded"). Such is the power of the mind that a dummy pill can be effective in up to 30 percent of cases. Hence a potential new treatment must be significantly better than the placebo treatment.

Some studies of alternative therapies in Asian countries, including China, India, and Thailand, appear to meet these standards. However, they get positive results essentially all the time, making them rather suspect to all but the most gullible.

Unfortunately, many therapies are touted as being beneficial to people with diabetes without a shred of scientific justification. In the next few questions we review some of the treatments that are often suggested as alternatives to conventional medications. For further information, the best and most comprehensive source about alternative treatments is HealthGate's "Natural Pharmacist," which is licensed to several Web sites.

99. I heard about a study of people with diabetes in China who benefited from taking large amounts of chromium. Would that help me?

All of us do need at least trace amounts of chromium in our diets. The most important thing that it does is regulate the amount of glucose in our blood by working with insulin.

There is evidence to suggest that some people may be deficient in chromium. Good sources of chromium, such as wheat, are stripped of their chromium when they are processed. The biggest problem is that we don't have a good test to identify chromium status or chromium deficiency.

There are some safety concerns, because chromium is a heavy metal that could build up if you take too much of it. But this is only a problem with one form of chromium, the hexavalent (i.e., six bonding sites) form that occurs as a contaminant in the environment. Chromium in food is in the trivalent form (i.e., three binding sites) and there is little evidence of toxicity. Chromium picolinate is the most common chromium supplement, but there are several health concerns about this form of the mineral. It might be harmful for individuals with depression, bipolar disease, or schizophrenia, and it might cause a severe skin reaction. However, the supplement is also available as chromium polynicotinate, chromium chloride, and high-chromium brewer's yeast.

The study of chromium supplementation in China is perhaps the best known. Researchers studied the effects of 1,000 micrograms of chromium, 200 micrograms of chromium, and a placebo (dummy pill) on 180 Chinese men and women with type 2 diabetes. After two months, their A1c values were much better in the groups that received 1,000 mcg, and after four months in both supplemented groups. While these results suggest a benefit from chromium supplementation, there is some speculation that the soil that yields the foods eaten by these people is depleted of chromium through intensive use, so that supplementation may only be of benefit when dietary intake is inadequate.

100. Is vanadium safe for people with diabetes to take as a blood glucose control?

Like chromium, vanadium is a mineral that has been recommended for people with diabetes and for body-builders. But even though we may need trace amounts of vanadium, anything above very low dosages can be danger-ous, and there is no conclusive evidence that it is effective.

Some animal studies indicate that vanadium might work like insulin to control blood glucose levels. Preliminary human studies indicate that it might have the same effect on people. But the margin between a therapeutic and a toxic dose is so small—probably less than for any other treatment for diabetes—that you should never consider vanadium unless you are under the careful supervision of a physician.

101. Will ginseng reduce my blood glucose levels? I've heard some varieties do but not others.

Three different plants are commonly called ginseng. The best known is probably Korean ginseng (Panax ginseng). Another type is American ginseng (Panax quinquefolius). But the so-called Siberian ginseng isn't ginseng at all.

One double-blind study of 100 mg to 200 mg Korean ginseng on 36 people with type 2 diabetes showed some improvement in their blood glucose levels. But even the authors say that it was probably because the ginseng group exercised more. Improved blood sugar control was also seen in two small double-blind placebo-controlled trials using American ginseng. But one study suggests that American ginseng with low ginsenoside content is not effective. More research is needed and is underway.

KEY TO THE TABLE

GI: The glycemic index for the food, where glucose equals 100

Nominal Serving Size: The portion of food tested

Net Carb per Serving: The total grams of carbs available to the body for digestion from the particular food in the specific serving size (total grams of carbs minus grams of fiber)

GL per Serving: Glycemic load of the food; this relates to the quantity of carbs that will enter the bloodstream for the particular food in the specific serving size

THE GLYCEMIC INDEX AND GLYCEMIC LOAD TABLE

The Table in this section will help you find a food's glycemic index quickly and easily, because we've listed the foods alphabetically.

The list provides not only the food's glycemic index but also its glycemic load (GL = carbohydrate content × GI ÷ 100). We calculate the glycemic load using a nominal, or standardized, serving size as well as the carbohydrate content of that serving—both of which we've also listed. That way, you can choose foods with either a low glycemic index or a low glycemic load. If your favorite food is both high GI and high GL, you can either cut down the serving size or dilute the GL by combining it with very low GI foods, such as rice and lentils.

For the first time, we've also included foods that have very little carbohydrate; their GI value is zero, indicated by [0]. Many vegetables, such as avocados and broccoli, and protein foods such as chicken, cheese, and tuna, fall into the low- or no-carbohydrate category. Most alcoholic beverages are also low in carbohydrate.

Food	GI Value per Serving	Nominal Serving Size	Net Carb per Serving	GL per Serving
A				
All-Bran®, breakfast cereal	34	½ cup	15	4
Almonds	[0]	1.75 oz	0	0
Angel food cake, 1 slice	67	⅛ cake	29	19
Apple, dried	29	9 rings (2 oz.)	34	10
Apple, fresh, medium	38	4 oz	15	6
Apple juice, unsweetened	40	8 oz	29	12
Apple muffin, small	46	2 oz	29	13
Apricots, canned in light syrup	64	4 halves	19	12
Apricots, dried	29	2 oz.	34	10
Apricots, fresh, 3 medium	57	6 oz	13	7
Arborio, risotto rice, cooked	69	¾ cup	43	29
Artichokes (Jerusalem)	[0]	½ cup	0	0
Avocado	[0]	¼	0	0
B				
Bagel, white	72	1	35	25
Baked beans	38	⅔ cup	31	12
Baked beans, canned in tomato sauce	49	½ cup	17	8
Banana cake, 1 slice	51	⅛ cake	38	18
Banana, fresh, medium	52	4 oz	26	13
Barley, pearled, cooked	25	1 cup	32	8
Basmati rice, white, cooked	58	1 cup	38	22
Beef	[0]	3 oz	0	0
Beer	66	8 oz	10	0
Beets, canned	64	½ cup	7	5
Bengal gram dhal, chickpea	11	5 oz	36	4
Black bean soup	64	1 cup	27	17
Black beans, cooked	30	¾ cup	25	5
Black-eyed peas, canned	42	⅔ cup	17	7
Blueberry muffin, small	59	2 oz	29	17
Bok choy, raw	[0]	½ cup	0	0
Bran Flakes™, breakfast cereal	74	¾ cup	18	13
Bran muffin, small	60	2 oz	24	15
Brandy	[0]	1 oz	0	0
Brazil nuts	[0]	1.75 oz	0	0
Breton wheat crackers	67	6 crackers	14	10
Broad beans	79	½ cup	11	9
Broccoli, raw	[0]	½ cup	0	0
Broken rice, white, cooked	86	1 cup	43	37
Brown rice, cooked	66	1 cup	37	24
Buckwheat	54	¾ cup	30	16
Bulgur, cooked 20 min	48	½ cup	26	12
Bun, hamburger	61	1 oz	15	9
Butter beans, canned	31	½ cup	20	6
C				
Cabbage, raw	[0]	½ cup	0	0

[0] indicates that the food has so little carbohydrate that the GI value cannot be tested. The GL, therefore, is 0.

Food	GI Value per Serving	Nominal Serving Size	Net Carb per Serving	GL per Serving
Cactus Nectar, Organic Agave, light, 90% fructose (Western Commerce)	11	1 Tbsp	8	1
Cactus Nectar, Organic Agave, light, 97% fructose (Western Commerce)	10	1 Tbsp	8	1
Cantaloupe, fresh	67	4 oz	6	4
Capellini pasta, cooked	45	1 cup	45	20
Carrot juice, fresh	43	8 oz	23	10
Carrots, peeled, cooked	41	½ cup	5	2
Carrots, raw	47	1 medium	6	3
Cashew nuts, salted	22	1 oz	9	2
Cauliflower, raw	[0]	½ cup	0	0
Celery, raw	[0]	2 stalks	0	0
Cheese	[0]	1 oz	0	0
Cherries, fresh	63	1 cup	12	3
Chicken nuggets, frozen	46	3.5 oz	16	7
Chickpeas, canned	40	½ cup	22	9
Chickpeas, dried, cooked	28	⅔ cup	30	8
Chocolate cake made from mix with chocolate frosting	38	3 oz	52	20
Chocolate milk, low fat	34	8 oz	26	9
Chocolate mousse, 2% fat	31	½ cup	22	7
Chocolate powder, dissolved in water	55	8 oz	16	9
Chocolate pudding, made from powder and whole milk	47	½ cup	24	11
Choice DM™, nutritional support product, vanilla (Mead Johnson)	23	8 oz	24	6
Clif® Bar (cookies & cream)	101	2.4 oz	34	34
Coca Cola®, soft drink	53	8 oz	26	14
Cocoa Puffs™, breakfast cereal	77	1 cup	26	20
Complete™, breakfast cereal	48	1 cup	21	10
Condensed milk, sweetened	61	2 oz	28	17
Converted rice, long-grain, cooked 20-30 min, Uncle Ben's	50	1 cup	36	18
Converted rice, white, cooked 20-30 min, Uncle Ben's	38	1 cup	36	14
Corn Flakes™, breakfast cereal	77	1 cup	25	20
Corn Flakes™, Honey Crunch, breakfast cereal	72	¾ cup	25	18
Cornmeal, cooked 2 min	68	⅔ cup	13	9
Corn pasta, gluten-free	78	1¼ cups	42	32
Corn Pops™, breakfast cereal	80	1 cup	26	21
Corn Thins, puffed corn cakes, gluten-free	87	1 oz	20	18
Corn, sweet, cooked	48	1 ear	16	8
Couscous, cooked 5 min	65	1 cup	33	21
Cranberry juice cocktail	52	8 oz	31	16
Crispix™, breakfast cereal	87	1 cup	25	22
Croissant, medium	67	2 oz	26	17
Cucumber, raw	[0]	½ cup	0	0
Cupcake, strawberry-iced, small	73	1.5 oz	26	19
Custard apple, raw, flesh only	54	4 oz	19	10

[0] indicates that the food has so little carbohydrate that the GI value cannot be tested. The GL, therefore, is 0.

Food	GI Value per Serving	Nominal Serving Size	Net Carb per Serving	GL per Serving
Custard, homemade	43	½ cup	17	7
Custard, prepared from powder with whole milk, instant	35	½ cup	26	9
D				
Dates, dried	39	2 oz	40	16
Desiree potato, peeled, cooked	101	5 oz	17	17
Doughnut, cake type	76	1.75 oz	23	17
E				
Eggs, large	[0]	2	0	0
Enercal Plus™ (Wyeth-Ayerst)	61	8 oz	40	24
English Muffin™ bread (Natural Ovens)	77	1 oz	14	11
Ensure™, vanilla drink	48	8 oz	34	16
Ensure™ bar, chocolate fudge brownie	43	1.4 oz	20	8
Ensure Plus™, vanilla drink	40	8 oz	47	19
Ensure Pudding™, old-fashioned vanilla	36	4 oz	26	9
F				
Fanta®, orange soft drink	68	8 oz	34	23
Fettuccine, egg, cooked	40	1 cup	46	18
Figs, dried	61	2 oz	26	16
Fish	[0]	3 oz	0	0
Fish sticks	38	3.5 oz	19	7
Flan/crème caramel	65	½ cup	73	47
French baguette, white, plain	95	1 oz	15	15
French fries, frozen, reheated in microwave	75	30 pcs	29	22
French green beans, cooked	[0]	½ cup	0	0
French vanilla cake made from mix, with vanilla frosting	42	3.5 oz	58	24
French vanilla ice cream, premium, 16% fat	38	½ cup	14	5
Froot Loops™, breakfast cereal	69	1 cup	26	18
Frosted Flakes™, breakfast cereal	55	¾ cup	26	15
Fructose, pure	19	1 Tbsp	10	2
Fruit cocktail, canned, light syrup	55	½ cup	16	9
Fruit leather	61	2 pcs	24	15
G				
Gatorade™ (orange) sports drink	78	8 oz	15	12
Gin	[0]	1 oz	0	0
Glucerna™, vanilla (Abbott)	31	8 oz	23	7
Glucose (dextrose)	99	1 Tbsp	10	10
Glucose tablets	102	3 pcs	15	15
Gluten-free corn pasta	76	1¼ cups	49	37
Gluten-free multigrain bread	79	1 oz	13	10
Gluten-free rice and corn pasta	76	1½ cups	49	37
Gluten-free spaghetti, rice and split pea, canned in tomato sauce	68	8 oz	27	19
Gluten-free split pea and soy pasta shells	29	1½ cups	31	9
Gluten-free white bread, sliced	80	1 oz	15	12

[0] indicates that the food has so little carbohydrate that the GI value cannot be tested. The GL, therefore, is 0.

Food	GI Value per Serving	Nominal Serving Size	Net Carb per Serving	GL per Serving
Glutinous (sticky) rice, white, cooked	98	¾ cup	32	31
Gnocchi	68	6 oz	48	33
Grapefruit juice, unsweetened	48	8 oz	22	9
Grapefruit, fresh, medium	25	1 half	11	3
Grape-Nuts® (Post), breakfast cereal	75	¼ cup	21	16
Grapes, black, fresh	59	¾ cup	18	11
Grapes, green, fresh	46	¾ cup	18	8
Green peas	48	½ cup	7	3
Green pea soup, canned	66	8 oz	41	27

H

Food	GI Value per Serving	Nominal Serving Size	Net Carb per Serving	GL per Serving
Hamburger bun	61	½ oz	15	9
Happiness™ (cinnamon, raisin, pecan bread) (Natural Ovens)	63	1 oz	14	9
Hazelnuts	[0]	1.75 oz	0	0
Healthy Choice™ Hearty 100% Whole Grain	62	1 oz	14	9
Healthy Choice™ Hearty 7-Grain	55	1 oz	14	8
Honey	55	1 Tbsp	18	10
Hot cereal, apple & cinnamon, dry (Con Agra)	37	1.2 oz	22	8
Hot cereal, unflavored, dry (Con Agra)	25	1.2 oz	19	5
Hunger Filler™, whole-grain bread (Natural Ovens)	59	1 oz	13	7

I

Food	GI Value per Serving	Nominal Serving Size	Net Carb per Serving	GL per Serving
Ice cream, low fat, vanilla, "light"	50	½ cup	9	5
Ice cream, premium, French vanilla, 16% fat	38	½ cup	14	5
Ice cream, premium, "ultra chocolate," 15% fat	37	½ cup	14	7
Ice cream, regular fat	61	½ cup	20	12
Instant potato, mashed	85	¾ cup	20	17
Instant rice, white, cooked 6 min	87	¾ cup	42	29
Ironman PR® bar, chocolate	39	2.3 oz	26	10

J

Food	GI Value per Serving	Nominal Serving Size	Net Carb per Serving	GL per Serving
Jam, apricot fruit spread, reduced sugar	55	1½ Tbsps	13	7
Jam, strawberry	46	1½ Tbsps	9	4
Jasmine rice, white, cooked	109	¾ cup	42	46
Jelly beans	78	1 oz	28	22

K

Food	GI Value per Serving	Nominal Serving Size	Net Carb per Serving	GL per Serving
Kaiser roll	73	1 half	16	12
Kavli™ Norwegian crispbread	71	5 pcs	16	12
Kidney beans, canned	52	⅔ cup	17	9
Kidney beans, cooked	23	⅔ cup	25	6
Kiwi fruit	53	4 oz	12	6
Kudos® Whole Grain Bars, chocolate chip	62	1.8 oz	32	20

L

Food	GI Value per Serving	Nominal Serving Size	Net Carb per Serving	GL per Serving
Lactose, pure	46	1 Tbsp	10	5
Lamb	[0]	3 oz	0	0
Leafy vegetables (spinach, arugula, etc.), raw	[0]	1½ cups	0	0
L.E.A.N Fibergy™ bar, Harvest Oat	45	1.75 oz	29	13

[0] indicates that the food has so little carbohydrate that the GI value cannot be tested. The GL, therefore, is 0.

Food	GI Value per Serving	Nominal Serving Size	Net Carb per Serving	GL per Serving
L.E.A.N Life long Nutribar™, Chocolate Crunch	32	1.5 oz	19	6
L.E.A.N Life long Nutribar™, Peanut Crunch	30	1.5 oz	19	6
L.E.A.N Nutrimeal™, drink powder, Dutch chocolate	26	8 oz	13	3
Lemonade, reconstituted	66	8 oz	20	13
Lentil soup, canned	44	8 oz	21	9
Lentils, brown, cooked	29	¾ cup	18	5
Lentils, green, cooked	30	¾ cup	17	5
Lentils, red, cooked	26	¾ cup	18	5
Lettuce	[0]	1 cup	0	0
Life Savers®, peppermint candy	70	18 pcs	30	21
Light rye bread	68	1 oz	14	10
Lima beans, baby, frozen	32	½ cup	30	10
Linguine pasta, thick, cooked	46	1 cup	48	22
Linguine pasta, thin, cooked	52	1 cup	45	23
Long-grain rice, cooked 10 min	50	¾ cup	41	23
Lychees, canned in syrup, drained	79	4 oz	20	16

M

Food	GI Value per Serving	Nominal Serving Size	Net Carb per Serving	GL per Serving
M & M's®, peanut	33	1 oz	17	6
Macadamia nuts	[0]	1.75 oz	0	0
Macaroni and cheese, made from mix	64	1¼ cup	51	32
Macaroni, cooked	47	1¼ cups	48	23
Maltose	105	1 Tbsp	10	11
Mango	51	4 oz	17	8
Maple syrup, pure Canadian	54	1 Tbsp	18	10
Marmalade, orange	55	1½ Tbsps	20	9
Mars Bar®	62	2 oz	40	25
Melba toast, Old London	70	6 pcs	23	16
METRx® bar (vanilla)	74	3.6 oz	50	37
Milk Arrowroot™ cookies	69	5	18	12
Millet, cooked	71	¾ cup	36	25
Mini Wheats™, whole-wheat breakfast cereal	58	12 pcs	21	12
Mousse, butterscotch, 1.9% fat	36	1.75 oz	10	4
Mousse, chocolate, 2% fat	31	1.75 oz	11	3
Mousse, hazelnut, 2.4% fat	36	1.75 oz	10	4
Mousse, mango, 1.8% fat	33	1.75 oz	11	4
Mousse, mixed berry, 2.2% fat	36	1.75 oz	10	4
Mousse, strawberry, 2.3% fat	32	1.75 oz	10	3
Muesli bar containing dried fruit	61	1 oz	21	13
Muesli bread, made from mix in bread oven (Con Agra)	54	1 oz	12	7
Muesli, gluten-free, with low-fat milk	39	1 oz	19	7
Muesli, Swiss Formula	56	1 oz	16	9
Muesli, toasted	43	1 oz	17	7
Multi-Grain 9-Grain bread	43	1 oz	14	6

N

Food	GI Value per Serving	Nominal Serving Size	Net Carb per Serving	GL per Serving
Navy beans, canned	38	5 oz	31	12
Nesquik™, chocolate dissolved in low-fat milk, no-sugar-added	41	8 oz	11	5

[0] indicates that the food has so little carbohydrate that the GI value cannot be tested. The GL, therefore, is 0.

Food	GI Value per Serving	Nominal Serving Size	Net Carb per Serving	GL per Serving
Nesquik™, strawberry dissolved in low-fat milk, no-sugar-added	35	8 oz	12	4
New creamer potato, canned	65	5 oz	18	12
New creamer potato, unpeeled and cooked 20 min	78	5 oz	21	16
Noodles, instant "two-minute" (Maggi®)	46	1½ cups	40	19
Noodles, mung bean (Lungkow beanthread), dried, cooked	39	1½ cups	45	18
Noodles, rice, fresh, cooked	40	1½ cups	39	15
Nutella®, chocolate hazelnut spread	33	1 Tbsp	12	4
Nutrigrain™, breakfast cereal	66	½ cup	15	10
Nutty Natural™, whole-grain bread (Natural Ovens)	59	1 oz	12	7
O				
Oat bran, raw	55	2 Tbsp	5	3
Oatmeal, cooked 1 min	66	1 cup	26	17
Oatmeal cookies	54	2 small	17	9
Orange juice, unsweetened, reconstituted	53	8 oz	18	9
Orange, fresh, medium	42	4 oz	11	5
P				
Pancakes, buckwheat, gluten-free, made from mix	102	1 pancake	22	22
Pancakes, prepared from mix	67	1 pancake	23	15
Papaya, fresh	56	4 oz	8	5
Parsnips	97	½ cup	12	12
Pastry	59	2 oz	26	15
Pea soup, canned	66	8 oz	41	27
Peach, canned in heavy syrup	58	½ cup	15	9
Peach, canned in light syrup	57	½ cup	18	9
Peach, fresh, large	38	4 oz	11	4
Peanuts	14	1.75 oz	6	1
Pear halves, canned in natural juice	44	½ cup	13	5
Pear, fresh	38	4 oz	11	4
Peas, green, frozen, cooked	48	½ cup	7	3
Pecans	10	1.75 oz	0	0
Pepper, fresh, green or red	[0]	½ cup	0	0
Pineapple juice, unsweetened	46	8 oz	34	16
Pineapple, fresh	59	¾ oz	10	6
Pinto beans, canned	45	⅔ cup	22	10
Pinto beans, dried, cooked	39	¾ cup	26	10
Pita bread, white	57	1 oz	17	10
Pizza, cheese	60	1 slice	27	16
Pizza, Super Supreme, pan (11.4% fat)	36	1 slice	24	9
Pizza, Super Supreme, thin and crispy (13.2% fat)	30	1 slice	22	7
Plums, fresh	39	1 medium	12	5
Pop Tarts™, double chocolate	70	1.8 oz pastry	36	25
Popcorn, plain, cooked in microwave oven	72	2 cups	11	8
Pork	[0]	3 oz	0	0
Potato chips, plain, salted	54	1.75 oz	18	10
Potato, baked	77	5 oz	30	23

[0] indicates that the food has so little carbohydrate that the GI value cannot be tested. The GL, therefore, is 0.

Food	GI Value per Serving	Nominal Serving Size	Net Carb per Serving	GL per Serving
Potato, microwaved	79	5 oz	18	14
Pound cake (Sara Lee)	54	1.75 oz	23	12
PowerBar® (chocolate)	57	2.3 oz	42	24
Premium soda crackers	74	5 crackers	17	12
Pretzels	83	1 oz	20	16
Prunes, pitted	29	2 oz	33	10
Pudding, instant, chocolate, made with whole milk	47	½ cup	16	7
Pudding, instant, vanilla, made with whole milk	40	½ cup	16	6
Puffed crispbread	81	1 oz	19	15
Puffed rice cakes, white	82	3 cakes	21	17
Puffed Wheat, breakfast cereal	80	2 cups	21	17
Pumpernickel rye kernel bread	41	1 oz	12	5
Pumpkin	75	½ cup	4	3
Q				
Quinoa, organic, boiled	53	¾ cup	17	9
R				
Raisin Bran™, breakfast cereal	73	½ cup	19	14
Raisins	64	½ cup	44	28
Ravioli, meat-filled, cooked	39	6 oz	38	15
Red wine	[0]	3.5 oz	0	0
Red-skinned potato, peeled and microwaved on high for 6–7.5 min	79	5 oz	18	14
Red-skinned potato, peeled, boiled 35 min	88	5 oz	18	16
Red-skinned potato, peeled, mashed	91	5 oz	20	18
Resource Diabetic™, nutritional support product, vanilla (Novartis)	34	8 oz	23	8
Rice and corn pasta, gluten-free	76	1¼ cups	49	37
Rice bran, extruded	19	1 oz	14	3
Rice cakes, white	82	1 oz	21	17
Rice Krispies Treat™ bar	63	1 oz	24	15
Rice Krispies™, breakfast cereal	82	1¼ cups	26	22
Rice noodles, fresh, cooked	40	1½ cups	39	15
Rice, parboiled	72	1 cup	36	26
Rice pasta, brown, cooked 16 min	92	1 cup	38	35
Rice vermicelli	58	1¼ cups	39	22
Rolled oats	42	1 cup	21	9
Roll-Ups®, processed fruit snack	99	1 oz	25	24
Roman (cranberry) beans, fresh, cooked	46	¾ cup	18	8
Russet, baked potato	77	5 oz	30	23
Rutabaga, fresh, cooked	72	5 oz	10	7
Rye bread	58	1 oz	14	8
Ryvita® crackers	69	3 crackers	16	11
S				
Salami	[0]	1 oz	0	0
Salmon	[0]	3 oz	0	0
Sausages, fried	28	3.5 oz	3	1
Scones, plain	92	1 oz	9	8

[0] indicates that the food has so little carbohydrate that the GI value cannot be tested. The GL, therefore, is 0.

Food	Serving	Size	Serving	Serving
Sebago potato, peeled, cooked	87	5 oz	17	14
Seeded rye bread	55	1 oz	13	7
Semolina, cooked	55	⅓ cup (dry)	50	28
Shellfish (shrimp, crab, lobster, etc.)	[0]	3 oz	0	0
Sherry	[0]	2 oz	0	0
Shortbread cookies	64	1 oz	16	10
Shredded Wheat™, breakfast cereal	75	½ cup	20	15
Shredded Wheat™ biscuits	62	1 oz	18	11
Skim milk	32	8 oz	12	4
Skittles®	70	45 pcs	45	32
Smacks™, breakfast cereal	71	¾ cup	23	11
Smoothie, raspberry (Con Agra)	33	8 oz	41	14
Snack bar, Apple Cinnamon (Con Agra)	40	1.75 oz	29	12
Snack bar, Peanut Butter & Choc-Chip (Con Agra)	37	1.75 oz	27	10
Snickers® bar	41	2 oz	36	15
Soda Crackers, Premium	74	5 crackers	17	12
Soft drink, Coca Cola®	53	8 oz	26	14
Soft drink, Fanta®, orange	68	8 oz	34	23
Sourdough rye	48	1 oz	12	6
Sourdough wheat	54	1 oz	14	8
Soy & Flaxseed bread (mix in bread oven) (Con Agra)	50	1 oz	10	5
Soybeans, canned	14	½ cup	6	1
Soybeans, dried, cooked	20	1 cup	6	1
Spaghetti, durum wheat, cooked 20 min	64	1½ cups	43	27
Spaghetti, gluten-free, rice and split pea, canned in tomato sauce	68	8 oz	27	19
Spaghetti, white, cooked 5 min	44	1 cups	48	21
Spaghetti, whole wheat, cooked 5 min	42	1¼ cups	42	16
Special K™, breakfast cereal	56	1 cup	21	11
Spirali pasta, durum wheat, al dente	43	1½ cups	44	19
Split pea and soy pasta shells, gluten-free	29	1½ cups	31	9
Split-pea soup	60	1 cup	27	16
Split peas, yellow, cooked 20 min	32	¾ cup	19	6
Sponge cake, plain	46	2 oz	36	17
Squash, raw	[0]	½ cup	0	0
Star pastina, white, cooked 5 min	38	1½ cups	48	18
Stay Trim™, whole-grain bread (Natural Ovens)	70	1 oz	15	10
Stoned Wheat Thins	67	14 crackers	17	12
Strawberries, fresh	40	1 cup	3	1
Strawberry jam	46	1½ Tbsps	9	4
Strawberry shortcake	42	2.2 oz	40	17
Stuffing, bread	74	½ cup	21	16
Sucrose	60	1 Tbsp	10	7
Super Supreme pizza, pan (11.4% fat)	36	1 slice	24	9
Super Supreme pizza, thin and crispy (13.2% fat)	30	1 slice	22	7
Sushi, salmon	48	3.5 oz	36	17
Sweet corn, whole kernel, canned, diet-pack, drained	46	⅓ cup	14	7
Sweet potato, cooked	46	5 oz	25	11

[0] indicates that the food has so little carbohydrate that the GI value cannot be tested. The GL, therefore, is 0.

Food	GI Value per Serving	Nominal Serving Size	Net Carb per Serving	GL per Serving
T				
Taco shells, baked	68	2 shells	12	8
Tapioca, cooked with milk	81	¾ cup	18	14
Tofu-based frozen dessert, chocolate with high-fructose (24%) corn syrup	115	1.75 oz	9	10
Tomato juice, canned, no added sugar	38	8 oz	9	4
Tomato soup	38	1 cup	17	6
Tortellini, cheese	50	6 oz	21	10
Tortilla chips, plain, salted	63	1.75 oz	26	17
Total™, breakfast cereal	76	¾ cup	22	17
Tuna	[0]	3 oz	0	0
Twix® Cookie Bar, caramel	44	2 cookies	39	17
U				
Ultracal™ with fiber (Mead Johnson)	40	8 oz	29	12
Ultra chocolate ice cream, premium, 15% fat	37	½ cup	14	5
V				
Vanilla cake made from mix, with vanilla frosting	42	3.5 oz	58	24
Vanilla pudding, instant, made with whole milk	40	½ cup	16	6
Vanilla wafers	77	7 cookies	18	14
Veal	[0]	3 oz	0	0
Vermicelli, white, cooked	35	1 cup	44	16
W				
Waffles, Aunt Jemima®	76	1 4″ waffle	13	10
Walnuts	[0]	1.75 oz	0	0
Water crackers	78	7 crackers	18	14
Watermelon, fresh	76	6 oz	6	4
Weet-Bix™, breakfast cereal	69	2 biscuits	17	12
Wheaties™, breakfast cereal	82	1 cup	21	17
Whiskey	[0]	1 oz	0	0
White bread	70	1 oz	14	10
White rice, instant, cooked 6 min	87	1 cup	42	36
White wine	[0]	3.5 oz	0	0
100% Whole Grain™ bread (Natural Ovens)	51	1 oz	13	7
Whole milk	31	8 oz	12	4
Whole-wheat bread	77	1 oz	12	9
Wonder™ white bread	80	1 oz	15	12
X				
Xylitol	8	1 Tbsp	10	1
Y				
Yam, peeled, cooked	37	5 oz	36	13
Yogurt, low fat, wild strawberry	31	8 oz	34	11
Yogurt, low fat, with fruit and artificial sweetener	14	8 oz	15	2
Yogurt, low fat, with fruit and sugar	33	8 oz	35	12

[0] indicates that the food has so little carbohydrate that the GI value cannot be tested. The GL, therefore, is 0.

GLOSSARY

A1C

A test that measures a person's average blood glucose level over the past 2 to 3 months. Also called hemoglobin A1c or glycosylated or glycated hemoglobin, the test indicates the percentage of hemoglobin that is "glycated," i.e. has a glucose molecule riding on its back. (Hemoglobin is the part of a red blood cell that carries oxygen to the cells and sometimes joins with the glucose in the bloodstream.) This is proportional to the amount of glucose in the blood.

ALPHA-GLUCOSIDASE INHIBITORS

A class of oral medicine for type 2 diabetes that blocks enzymes that digest sugars and starches in food. When these medicines are used, the rise in blood glucose levels is slower and lower after meals. Side effects may include flatulence and diarrhea, but the dose can be titrated to minimize symptoms. Generic names: acarbose and miglitol.

AMYLOPECTIN

A type of starch consisting of highly branched glucose-based polysaccharides of high molecular weight. Amylopectin molecules are larger and more open than amylose molecules, making the starch easier to cook and digest, so they have higher GI values than high-amylose starches. Waxy starches, such as waxy rice and waxy corn, are 100 percent amylopectin. But most starches are 70 to 80 percent amylopectin and 20 to 30 percent amylose (see amylose).

AMYLOSE

A type of starch consisting of straight chain glucose-based polysaccharides with unbranched, linear, or spiral structures. Amylose molecules form tight compact clumps that are harder to cook and digest than amylopectin molecules, so they have lower GI values than high-amylopectin starches. Some varieties of corn and rice contain up to 60 percent amylose.

ANTI-NUTRIENTS

A wide variety of substances present naturally in foods that are able to bind enzymes or nutrients and thereby block the action or absorption of nutrients. Tannin is a common anti-nutrient that blocks the absorption of iron. Uncooked legumes contain significant quantities of substances that block the absorption of protein and starch and compounds that can damage red cells (hemoglutins). This means that thorough cooking of legumes is essential.

BIGUANIDES

A class of oral medicine used to treat type 2 diabetes that lowers blood glucose by reducing the amount of glucose produced by the liver and by helping the body respond better to insulin. Generic name: metformin.

CARBOHYDRATE

One of the three main nutrients in food. Foods that are rich in carbohydrate are cereals and cereal products including bread, cookies, pasta, some vegetables (particularly potatoes, sweet potatoes, and sweet corn), most fruits, dairy products (except cheese), sugar, honey, jam, and candy.

CAROTENOIDS

Any of a class of yellow to orange pigments in foods, particularly in fruits and vegetables, including carotenes and xanthophylls. They are precursors of vitamin A and recognized as powerful antioxidants.

CORTISOL

A steroid hormone produced by the adrenal cortex that is involved in the regulation of carbohydrate metabolism. Since the body releases it when stressed or in an agitated state, cortisol has gained widespread attention as the so-called "stress hormone."

THE DAWN PHENOMENON

The early-morning (4 a.m. to 8 a.m.) rise in blood glucose level.

DEXTROSE

Also called glucose. The simple sugar found in blood that serves as the body's main source of energy.

DISACCHARIDE

A sugar formed from two single sugar molecules. For example, sucrose, which is composed of glucose and fructose. Lactose and maltose are also disaccharides.

FREE FOODS

Those foods that are essentially free of any impact on your blood sugar, for example meat and lettuce.

FRUCTOSE

Also known as fruit sugar or levulose. A sugar that occurs naturally in fruits and honey. Fructose consumption has a minor impact on blood glucose levels (GI = 20). In the liver, it is oxidized immediately to energy or slowly converted to glucose. Unlike glucose, it doesn't stimulate the production of insulin.

GALACTOSE

A sugar found in certain plant gums and mucilages, and one of the principal constituents of lactose, which is the main sugar in milk. Galactose is never found in free form in foods. Once in the liver galactose is slowly converted to glucose.

GLUCAGON

A hormone produced by the pancreas that raises the blood sugar level by promoting the conversion of glycogen to glucose in the liver (see glycogen).

GLUCOSE

A monosaccharide sugar widely present in most plant and animal tissue. It is the principal circulating sugar in the blood and the major energy source of the body.

GLYCEMIC INDEX

A ranking of carbohydrate exchanges in foods according to their immediate impact on blood glucose levels. To make a fair comparison, all foods are compared with a reference food such as pure glucose in equivalent carbohydrate amounts.

GLYCEMIC LOAD

A measure of the glycemic impact of foods based on both the type and amount of carbohydrate. It is calculated by multiplying the glycemic index of a food by the available carbohydrate content (carbohydrates minus fiber) in a serving (expressed in grams), divided by 100.

GLYCOGEN

The name given to glucose stores in the body. Glycogen can be readily broken down to glucose to maintain a normal blood glucose concentration. In an adult male, approximately two thirds of the body's glycogen is found in the muscles and one third in the liver. The total stores of glycogen are relatively small however, and will be exhausted in about 24 hours during starvation.

HYPOGLYCEMIA

A condition that occurs when one's blood glucose is lower than normal, usually less than 70 mg/dl. Signs include hunger, nervousness, shakiness, perspiration, dizziness or light-headedness, sleepiness, and confusion. If left untreated, hypoglycemia may lead to unconsciousness. Hypoglycemia is treated by consuming a carbohydrate-rich food such as a glucose tablet. It may also be treated with an injection of glucagon, if the person is unconscious or unable to swallow. Also called an insulin reaction.

INSULIN

A hormone that helps the body use glucose for energy. The beta cells of the pancreas make insulin. When the body cannot make enough insulin, insulin is taken by injection or through use of an insulin pump.

INSULIN RESISTANCE

If you have insulin resistance, your muscle and liver cells are not good at taking up glucose unless there's a lot of insulin about. Chances are you'll have very high insulin levels even in the fasting state, but particularly after a meal, when the body is trying hard to metabolize the carbohydrate in the meal.

INSULIN SENSITIVITY

If you are insulin sensitive, your muscle and liver cells take up glucose rapidly without the need for a whole lot of insulin. Exercise keeps you insulin sensitive; so does a moderately high carbohydrate intake.

KETOACIDOSIS

An emergency condition that can occur in people with type 1 diabetes. High blood glucose levels, along with a severe lack of insulin, cause breakdown of body fat for energy and results in the production of ketones at a rate greater than the body can metabolize them. Their accumulation in the blood interferes with the body's pH balance. Signs of ketoacidosis are nausea and vomiting, stomach pain, fruity breath odor, and rapid breathing. Untreated ketoacidosis can lead to coma and death.

KETOSIS

A condition in which the liver produces ketones as a fuel source from free fatty acids. It is a normal physiological response to starvation or a low carbohydrate diet. In people with type 1 diabetes, where there is a severe lack of insulin, it may lead to diabetic ketoacidosis. Signs of ketosis are nausea, vomiting, and stomach pain.

KETONES

A by-product from the breakdown of fat, which some cells can use for energy. The brain can use these instead of glucose when it is hard-pressed. Ketones are strong acids, and when the rate of production is greater than their rate of removal, their increased concentration in the blood will disrupt the body's acid-base balance.

LACTOSE

The sugar naturally found in milk. When digested by the enzyme lactase, it yields glucose and galactose. Many older children and adults lack the gut enzyme needed to digest lactose and may experience symptoms of stomach pain and diarrhea after consumption of milk. But cheese, yogurt, and other fermented dairy products can be consumed without a problem.

MALTODEXTRIN

A partially digested starch consisting of glucose monomers linked in multiples of three to six. Used as a food additive, primarily as a thickener, and to modify the texture of foods. It is not sweet to the taste.

MALTOSE

A disaccharide consisting of two glucose units and formed during the digestion of starch. Also called malt sugar.

MEGLITINIDES

A class of oral medicine for type 2 diabetes that lowers blood glucose by helping the pancreas make more insulin immediately after meals. Generic name: repaglinide.

OSMOTIC PRESSURE

Like balls that naturally roll downhill, molecules tend to move from areas of high concentration to areas of low concentration. If there is a semi-permeable barrier to movement (such as a cell membrane) then the pressure exerted on the barrier is called "osmotic" pressure. The formal definition is: the pressure exerted by the flow of water through a semipermeable membrane separating two solutions with different concentrations of solute. Osmotic pressure is a characteristic of all living cells.

PRE-DIABETES

A condition in which blood glucose levels are higher than normal, but are not high enough for a diagnosis of diabetes. People with pre-diabetes are at increased risk for developing type 2 diabetes and immediate heart disease and stroke. Other names for pre-diabetes are impaired glucose tolerance and impaired fasting glucose.

SATIETY

The state of feeling pleasantly full after eating. Some foods are more satiating than others.

THE SOMOGYI EFFECT

When the blood glucose level swings high following hypoglycemia. The Somogyi effect may follow an untreated hypoglycemic episode during the night and is caused by the release of stress hormones.

SUCROSE

A disaccharide or double sugar consisting of glucose and fructose. Known as table sugar or white sugar, it is found naturally in most fruits and in sugar cane and sugar beets.

SULFONYLUREAS

A class of oral medicine for type 2 diabetes that lowers blood glucose by helping the pancreas make more insulin and by helping the body better use the insulin it makes. Generic names: acetohexamide, chlorpropamide, glimepiride, glipizide, glyburide, tolazamide, tolbutamide.

SYNDROME X

Also called the metabolic syndrome. The tendency of several conditions to occur together, including obesity, insulin resistance, elevated blood glucose levels, hypertension, high triglycerides levels, and low levels of the good cholesterol (HDL). People with Syndrome X are often unaware that they are at high risk of heart attack.

THIAZOLIDINEDIONES

A class of oral medicine for type 2 diabetes that helps insulin take glucose from the blood into the cells for energy by making cells more sensitive to insulin. Generic names: pioglitazone and rosiglitazone.

TYPE 1 DIABETES

A condition characterized by high blood glucose levels caused by a total lack of insulin. It occurs when the body's immune system attacks the insulin-producing beta cells in the pancreas and destroys them. The pancreas then produces little or no insulin. Type 1 diabetes develops most often in young people but can appear in adults.

TYPE 2 DIABETES

A condition characterized by high blood glucose levels caused by an insufficiency of insulin and the body's inability to use insulin efficiently. Type 2 diabetes develops most often in middle-aged and older adults but can appear in young people.

ACKNOWLEDGMENTS

We'd like to thank Matthew Lore, our exacting and tireless publisher at Marlowe & Company/Avalon; Philippa Sandall, our talented and skillful literary agent in Sydney; and John Miller, Jonathan Powell, and Catherine Nord, our supportive and truly long-suffering spouses.

INDEX

A

A1c, 122, 189
acidic foods, 143–44
activity level, 22–23
AGEs (advanced glycated endproducts), 19–20
aging process, 19–20
alcoholic beverages, 23, 133–34
alpha-glucosidase inhibitors, 85, 165, 189
alternative therapies, 168–73
Alzheimer's disease, 20
amylopectin, 74, 77, 189–90
amylose, 77, 190
anti-nutrients, 139, 190
apricots, 151
aspartame, 132

B

barley, 138
bean salad, 141
berries, 46
beta-carotene, 95
biguanides, 164–65, 190
black pepper, 149
blood glucose levels
    alcohol's effect on, 23, 133–34
    causes of high, 1–2
    dairy products' effect on, 117–18
    danger of high, 12–13, 19–20
    danger of low, 14–15
    effect of sickness on, 103
    exercise's effect on, 162–63
    factors that affect, 22–23
    fat's effect on, 112–13, 119–20
    fiber's effect on, 125
    lowering, 2, 111, 160–61
    medications' effect on, 24, 105
    morning, 106–7
    normal, 9–11
    protein's effect on, 114–16, 119–20
    ranges of, 11
    stress and, 104
    testing, 17–18
    time between eating and rise in, 16
    weight gain and, 100–2
    worst foods for raising, 71–72
blood glucose meters, 17
brain function, low blood glucose and, 14–15, 21
breads, 54, 75–76

C

calories, 83
cancer, 66
candy, 91
cane sugar, 86
carbohydrates
    absorption of, 40–41
    available, 39, 61
    complex vs. simple, 25–26
    content of, in food, 29–30
    defined, 190
    fat with, 115–16
    glucose levels and, 9, 22
    with low GI values, 137–38
    on nutrition labels, 49
    protein with, 115–16
    serving sizes of, 27–28
carotenoids, 52, 94–95, 191
carrots, 140
cashews, 157
cereals, 48, 54, 84
cheese, 117, 156
cherries, 152
chickpeas, 141
chromium, 170–71
cinnamon, 148–49
coffee, 130

determining, 42–43
objectivity of, 65
glycogen, 9, 192

H

HbA1c, 122, 189
health benefits, of low-
GI diet, 66–67
health problems
associated with high
blood glucose levels,
12–13, 19–20
associated with low
blood glucose levels,
14–15
heart problems, 19, 66
high-fructose corn
syrup, 89, 92–93
honey, 85, 92
hypoglycemia, 14, 18,
135, 192–93

I

ice cream, 117, 156
illness, 103
infections, 22
insoluble fiber, 126
insulin
defined, 193
effects of, 66–67
function of, 2, 9–10
sensitivity, 27
taking, 166–67
insulin resistance
defined, 193
fasting and, 135
fat and, 112–13
low carbohydrate diet
and, 121–22
weight gain and,
100–2
insulin resistance
syndrome. See
Syndrome X
insulin sensitivity, 193
iron deficiency anemia,
139

J

Jerusalem artichokes,
50–51

jicama, 51

K

kamut, 50
ketoacidosis, 13, 101,
193–94
ketones, 13, 163, 194
ketosis, 163, 194

L

lactose, 92, 194
legumes, 16, 53, 139
lemon juice, 143–44
liver, 1, 9
Low Insulin Diet, 149
low-carbohydrate diets,
123

M

macadamia nuts, 51
maltodextrins, 80–82,
194
maltose, 80, 194
medications
effect of, on blood
glucose levels, 24,
105
to lower blood
glucose, 161,
164–65
meglitinides, 164, 195
menstrual cycle, 23
mental performance. See
brain function
metabolic syndrome,
19–20
milk, 117–18
mixed meals, 127–28
molasses, 86
mood swings, 21

N

new potatoes, 73–75
noncaloric sweeteners,
132
nopal, 145
nutrition labels
carbohydrate content
on, 49
glycemic index (GI)
and, 53

nuts, 50–51, 154,
157–58

O

oatmeal, 96, 138
obesity
diabetes and, 102
sugar consumption
and, 87
omega-3 fatty acids,
124, 157
osmotic pressure, 80–81,
195
overweight, 20

P

pain, 22
partially hydrogenated
oil, 97–98
pasta, 53, 137
peanuts, 157
phytoestrogens, 139
pineapple juice, 150
popcorn, 97, 137
porridge, 96, 138
portion sizes
glycemic index values
and, 42–44
glycemic load and, 65
moderation in, 71–72
potatoes
blood glucose levels
and, 71, 73–75, 142
sweet, 94–95
pre-diabetes, 19, 195
prednisone, 105
pregnancy, 23
premenstrual symptoms,
21
prickly pear cactus,
145
protein
in diet, 121–22
glycemic effect of,
50–51, 54, 115–16
long-term effect of,
119–20
pumpkin, 51–52

Q

quinoa, 50